The Harvest Collection

A Vegetarian Cookbook for All Seasons

Gardner Merchant

Avery Publishing Group

Garden City Park, New York

Cover Design: William Gonzalez
Editors: Alison Leach and Joanne Abrams

Library of Congress Cataloging-in-Publication Data
The Harvest collection: a vegetarian cookbook for all seasons/
  Gardner Merchant
     p.   cm.
  Includes index.
  ISBN 0-89529-615-2
    1. Vegetarian cookery.   I. Gardner Merchant (Firm)
  TX837.H374 1994
  641.5'636—dc20   93—45329
                                     CIP

Printed in the United States of America

10 9 8 7 6 5 4 3 2

Contents

Foreword v

Introduction 1

Nutritional Analysis 2

Cooking Peas and Beans 3

Culinary Tips 5

A Variety of Vegetarian Recipes
   The Spring Collection 8
   The Summer Collection 30
   The Autumn Collection 52
   The Winter Collection 74

Sauce Recipes 96

Garnishes for Different Seasons 99

Vegetarian Sandwiches 100

Glossary of Terms 102

Index 104

Foreword

Almost every time we open up a newspaper or magazine, we read about new scientific evidence which confirms that in one respect at least, our mothers were right all along. Vegetables *are* good for us. Unfortunately, a lot of people do not like vegetables regardless of the number of articles they read about preventing cancer and heart disease. And it's easy to understand why. Most of us grew up on vegetables that began canned or frozen and then were overcooked to mush, drenched in butter, and laden with salt. Later, we tasted the typical unseasoned vegetables available in most "good" restaurants. Although these vegetables were served hot, they were often undercooked to the point of being raw. No wonder vegetables are less popular than hamburgers!

Vegetarians like me have known for years that you can give up meat and processed foods without giving up pleasure. On the contrary, we have discovered wonderful tastes, textures, and aromas that people stuck in the meat-and-potatoes rut never dreamed of. The secret is in the preparation, the seasoning, and the presentation of the dishes. When these three aspects of cooking get the attention they deserve, even a simple meal of beans and rice can be transformed from ordinary to extraordinary. *The Harvest Collection* proves this, recipe after recipe. In each dish, healthy, whole foods are used to create an entrée or side dish that can be proudly served to anyone, from the confirmed vegetarian to the most discriminating gourmet to the picky eater who claims not to like vegetables. Each dish presented in *The Harvest Collection* is so beautifully composed and so creatively garnished that just looking at the pictures is enough to make you hungry. The recipes are also expertly seasoned with a wide range of herbs and spices. When food is this appealing, there is no need to even mention that it's healthy. The healthful qualities of the dish can remain the secret of the cook.

The recipes in this book are grouped into seasons, which is an excellent idea. To get the most out of any recipe in terms of both health and taste, it is important to use only the finest quality ingredients. And the only way to get high quality produce is to grow or buy it in season. Imported, out-of-season produce is always disappointing, even when it looks good. We have all eaten those hard, tasteless tomatoes that are sold in the winter. Even the most skillful chef can't make these taste good.

Most of the recipes in *The Harvest Collection* include suggestions for variations. Using these variations, you can change recipes to suit your own tastes. And as you become accustomed to making dishes in more than one way, you will learn to introduce your *own* variations. For instance, you'll find that different vegetables can be substituted for one another, and that most grains can be replaced by a different grain, depending on the recipe and on your own preferences. For example, millet or even pasta can often be substituted for rice. To lighten up a recipe that contains dairy products, low-fat soy milk can always be substituted for cow's milk with excellent results. When eggs are used in a recipe as a binding ingredient, you can always use a vegetarian egg substitute or two egg whites instead.

So let's get started. Turn to the section of the book that has recipes for the current season. Choose a dish that appeals to you, and go to the market to find the best quality ingredients available. Then take your beautiful, healthful produce home and start cooking. The results will be so good that you won't have to say, "Eat it. It's good for you." The food will talk for itself.

Vicki Rae Chelf
Author of the *Arrowhead Mills Cookbook*

Introduction

Designed to appeal to vegetarians and semi-vegetarians alike, this collection of recipes is far removed from the traditional image of vegetarian food being stodgy and dull. It shows how light, imaginative and appetizing it can be.

A selection of recipes has been made for each of the four seasons – spring, summer, autumn and winter – all emphasizing the potential of vegetarian cooking. Most of the recipes contain suggestions for variations, thus greatly extending the number of dishes for you to try.

A healthy, well-balanced diet is of course very important for everyone and this was carefully considered in choosing the recipes. Guidelines are given on how to achieve this simply, and each recipe is graded in terms of its protein, fat and fiber contents. Low-fat milk, low-fat cheeses, polyunsaturated fats and wholemeal flour are recommended as ingredients (where applicable).

Many people are still rather confused by the range of beans and peas that are now available in both supermarkets and health food shops. The use of the different types is simplified by the inclusion of a table setting out the exact preparation and cooking methods.

Vegetarian food is sometimes accused of being bland. The recipes will show you how the less pronounced flavors of beans and lentils can easily be enhanced by the subtle use of herbs, spices and accompanying sauces. Whenever possible, use fresh herbs; many varieties can be grown successfully in pots on a sunny windowsill or patio.

The color photographs of each dish show how important presentation is in making food look tempting. The garnishes are relatively simple and quick to make – they are, however, merely suggestions to stimulate your imagination. Even if you do not always have the time when making a dish for the family to add any garnish, try to do so when you are entertaining. Many of the recipes are ideal for introducing your friends to a healthier eating pattern – even those who have previously dismissed vegetarian dishes will be converted once they have tasted some of the gourmet treats in this book.

Many dishes are enhanced by an accompanying sauce; the recipes on pages 96–98 show how to make these taste wonderful without resorting to cream.

Apart from the recipes, you will find much invaluable information in this book. You may, for example, have to make sandwiches regularly and be in need of new ideas for fillings. From the thirty suggestions given on pages 100 and 101 you are certain to discover some combinations that will appeal to you. You will also find that the collection of culinary tips on page 5 will help you to achieve perfect results when following the recipes.

The Harvest Collection will certainly prove an indispensable source of inspiration to every health-conscious cook.

Unless otherwise stated each recipe serves 4.

Nutritional Analysis

For a healthy, well-balanced vegetarian diet it is important to consider the protein, fat and fiber content of any dish. *The Harvest Collection* offers an insight to the nutritional balance of each recipe.

It is recommended that a balanced vegetarian diet have sufficient protein and be low in fat and high in fiber. You will find some of the dishes included in this collection high in fat, some low in protein and others low in fiber. By choosing complementary dishes to eat at this meal, you can adjust the balance as necessary. *It must be emphasized that the analyses were calculated on the given ingredients; any variation will make the relevant analysis invalid.*

Protein

It is recommended that 13 percent of our total calories each day should come from protein. For someone consuming 2000 calories per day, this is the equivalent of 22 grams of protein eaten at each of the three meals. A meat eater would easily obtain 28 grams of protein from a 4-ounce portion of meat. Vegetarians, however, need to plan the entire meal carefully to ensure a good intake of protein. If the main dish is low in protein, choose complementary items with a high-protein level.

High-protein foods include soy products, beans, peas, wholegrains and seeds. Milk and cheese are also rich in protein but should be eaten in moderation because of their high level of saturated fat. Low-fat milk and low-fat cheeses are a healthier choice. Good sources of protein for vegetarians are:

Grains	wholegrain bread, pasta, rice, breakfast cereals, oats, rye and barley
Nuts and Seeds	cashews, hazelnuts, almonds, peanuts, sunflower seeds, sesame seeds
Peas and Beans	dried beans (eg: kidney, butter and haricot), lentils, chickpeas

Fat

It is recommended that 30 percent or less of our total daily calories come from fat. Most of us eat more than this. A balanced diet should contain some fat, and the occasional high-fat dish is not harmful, provided it is complemented by low-fat dishes. It is the overall balance over a period of time that is important, rather than a dish-by-dish or even meal-by-meal assessment.

Cholesterol

If you are concerned about your blood cholesterol levels, you should take care not to eat too much fat, particularly saturated fat. It is the total fat in your diet which can lead to a raised blood cholesterol level.

Fiber

The recommended intake is 30 grams of fiber per day. This is not difficult to achieve when you realize that on average one piece of fresh fruit contains 4 grams and one slice of wholemeal bread 3 grams. A diet high in fiber is considered to be beneficial to general health. A vegetarian diet naturally provides a high-fiber intake with its extensive use of fresh vegetables, wholemeal flours, grains and beans.

All these facts and figures may be difficult to absorb, so each recipe in this book has been analyzed for protein, fat and fiber and then given a grading of high, medium or low. These gradings are based on United States recommendations at the time of publication. The analyses relate to one portion based on the recommended portion yield from the relevant recipes.

	High	Medium	Low
Protein	17 g or more	12–16 g	0–11 g
Fat	18 g or more	6–17 g	0–5 g
Fiber	8 g or more	4–7g	0–3 g

Cooking Peas and Beans

Peas and beans are important ingredients in vegetarian cookery being good sources of protein and fiber but low in fat. Beans have a built-in protection system to prevent their being taken by "wildlife" in their natural environment. It is for this reason that they must be handled correctly before being used in recipes.

Wash dried peas or beans two or three times in fresh cold water, then drain. Cover with twice their volume of fresh cold water and allow to soak for a minimum of 4 hours or preferably overnight. Drain.

Put the peas or beans in a pot and cover with fresh cold water, bring to a boil and boil rapidly for 10 minutes. Reduce the heat, cover the pan and simmer until tender. (Actual cooking times shown in table.) If a pea or bean is cooked, it should squash easily when pressed. Lentils will form a pulp-like mixture.

Do not add salt, vinegar, lemon juice or any sauce or dressing until the peas or beans are cooked; otherwise you will find that their skins will toughen.

A pressure cooker can be used which will considerably reduce the cooking times. Consult the manufacturer's instruction booklet for details.

A number of the recipes in this book contain various types of peas and beans. All can be bought dried and the table below gives instructions as to the preparation and cooking requirements of each one after initial boiling. If these seem too time-consuming, the majority are also widely available canned.

PEA/BEAN	DESCRIPTION	PREPARATION	AVERAGE COOKING TIME
ADUKI BEANS	Small red beans with a sweet nutty taste; ideal addition to soups, stews, curries, salads and rice	Soak overnight	40 minutes
BLACK-EYED PEAS	Round white beans distinguished by a black mark on one side; use in soups, salads, rice dishes and casseroles	Soak overnight	45–50 minutes
BLACK BEANS	Shiny black beans mainly used for sprouting; use whole in savory dishes	Soak overnight	50–60 minutes
BROAD BEANS	Large flat brown beans, also known as fava, haba or horse bean; use in stews and casseroles	Soak overnight	1½ hours
BUTTER BEANS	Also known as lima beans, with a slightly sweet taste; blend well with most dishes	Soak overnight	1–1½ hours

CANNELLINI BEANS	Large white beans with a light texture	Soak overnight	45–50 minutes
CHICKPEAS	High in protein, a versatile bean with a unique taste, also known as garbanzo beans; use in falafel, hummus or can be added to most main courses and salads	Soak overnight	1–1½ hours
FLAGEOLET BEANS	Pale green beans usually cooked and puréed	Soak overnight	40–45 minutes
FUL MEDAME BEANS	Small brown beans, also known as Egyptian brown beans, with thick skins and earthy taste; use in soups and stews	Soak overnight	55–60 minutes
GREEN PEAS	Whole: pale green wrinkled skin; use in stews and hotpots. Split: usually cooked and puréed for use in soups	Soak overnight Soaking improves texture but can be cooked without	1–1½ hours 30 minutes
HARICOT BEANS	Small white beans often used to make baked beans, very high in protein and extremely versatile	Soak overnight	1½ hours
LENTILS	Vary in color from green, orange pink to brown, the most common being red; a valuable source of protein; use in a variety of dishes	Soaking is not necessary for red lentils; a short soaking period improves texture of other types	Red lentils 20 minutes Others 45 minutes
MUNG BEANS	Range in color from green through yellow to golden and black; olive green variety usually used for sprouting	Soak overnight	30–45 minutes
PINTO BEANS	A variety of haricot bean with a mottled brown skin which changes to pink when cooked	Soak overnight	1–1½ hours
RED KIDNEY BEANS	Plump, red and shiny; a classic ingredient in Mexican cooking but will add color and taste to most dishes	Soak overnight (essential)	1 hour
SOY BEANS	Very valuable source of protein, after cooking can be used in many foods; also available in commercial products, eg: soy milk, tofu, soy sauce and soy flour	Soak overnight	3 hours

Culinary Tips

This collection of tips, compiled during the testing of the recipes, will help you to achieve perfect results.

Remember always to use vegetable stock in all vegetarian recipes. Dilute one vegetable stock cube with 13 ounces of water or crumble the cube as specified in the recipes.

For recipes that involve stuffing peppers, always blanch the pepper first. The best method is to slice off the base thinly to allow the water to penetrate inside. Dip the pepper in boiling water for 1–2 minutes, remove and refresh in cold water. Slice off the top of the "lid" and reserve. Remove the seeds and discard.

In making hot yogurt sauce, use half yogurt, half Béchamel; this will help to prevent the yogurt from separating. (See page 96 for the Béchamel Sauce recipe.)

Where wholemeal flour is used in recipes, a mixture of 50 percent wholemeal flour and 50 percent white flour may be used to give a lighter texture. To enhance the appearance and quality of a dish, white sauces have been prepared with white flour.

The use of fresh herbs is recommended – you will find that their delicate flavors greatly improve a dish. If they are unavailable, dried herbs can be used but the quantities given in the recipes should be halved.

To make a bread basket for garnish, mold a triangle of bread into a suitable round container such as a dariole mold (see page 102). Place in a cool oven and bake until dry. Remove the basket, allow to cool and use as described.

To make filo pastry baskets, cut filo pastry into three 2-inch squares. Grease the outside of a dariole mold, lay one layer of filo on top and brush with water. Place a second layer of filo on top and brush with water; repeat with a third layer. Put the mold upside-down in the oven and bake at 400°F until golden, about 5–8 minutes. Carefully remove the pastry basket from the mold. This is an effective way to serve dressings.

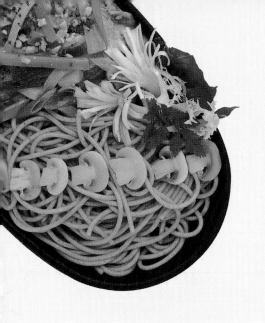

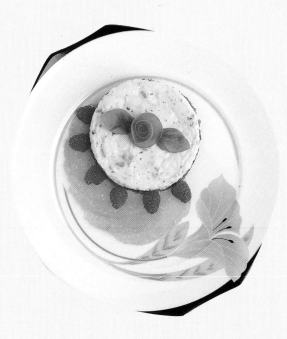

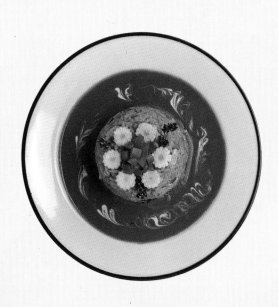

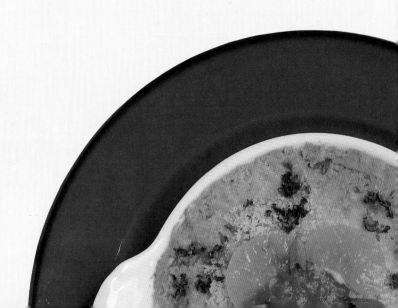

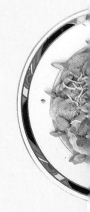

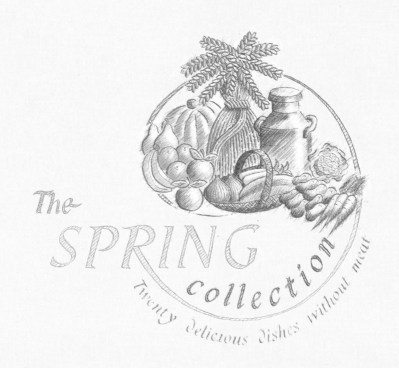

The
SPRING
collection

Twenty delicious dishes without meat

Hot Crudite!

2½ cups	cauliflower florets
Batter Mixture	
1 egg	
1 cup	low-fat milk
½ cup	flour
pinch salt	
Garlic Sauce	
1 cup	low-fat milk
1 onion clouté (see page 102)	
2 tbsp	polyunsaturated margarine
1 clove garlic, finely chopped	
2 tbsp	flour
salt and freshly ground pepper	
1–2 tsp	chopped fresh parsley

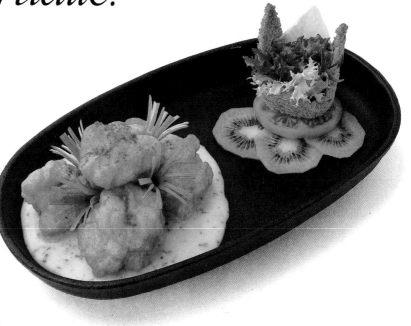

Cook the cauliflower in boiling water, until just tender but still firm. Drain well and refresh in cold water.

To make the batter, gradually blend the egg and milk with the flour and salt until a smooth mixture is formed. Dip the cauliflower in the batter and deep-fry in hot fat until crisp and golden brown. Drain thoroughly.

To make the garlic sauce, heat the milk with the onion clouté. Melt the margarine in a pan, stir in the garlic and sauté. Add the flour and make a roux (see page 103). Remove the onion and add the milk gradually, stirring constantly to make a smooth sauce. Allow the sauce to cook. Season and add the chopped parsley.

Arrange in a serving dish with a small quantity of garlic sauce as a coulis (see page 102). Serve the remaining sauce separately.

Variations
Use other vegetables, such as eggplant, zucchini or mushrooms, instead of the cauliflower.

Experiment with different sauces or dips, such as blue cheese sauce or yogurt and cucumber, instead of the garlic sauce.

Garnish scallion fleuron (see page 99); paprika; bread basket (see page 5); chicory leaf; red leaf lettuce; endive; fresh thyme; sliced tomato; kiwi fruit

Protein – low
Fat – medium
Fiber – medium

Cashew Paella

1 tbsp   polyunsaturated oil
1 medium onion, chopped
1 clove garlic, finely chopped
½ cup   brown rice
½ cup   long-grain rice
¾ cup   cashew nuts
1 tsp   paprika
1 tsp   chopped fresh basil
1 tsp   turmeric
½ red pepper, chopped
½ green pepper, chopped
2 stalks celery, chopped
2 cups   canned tomatoes, chopped
1½ cups   vegetable stock
salt and freshly ground pepper

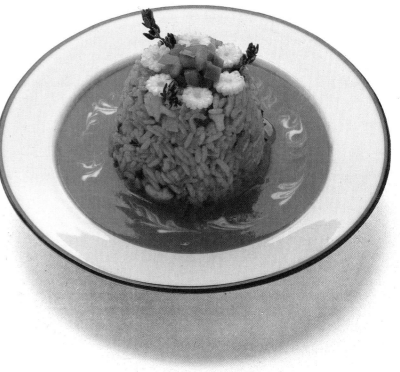

Heat the oil and sauté the onion and garlic until soft. Add both types of rice, the cashew nuts, paprika, basil and turmeric, and cook for 2 minutes. Then add the peppers, celery, tomatoes, stock, salt, and pepper. Simmer until the rice is just cooked – about 30 minutes.

Press the mixture into individual pudding molds, and turn out onto plates. Serve with tomato sauce (see page 96).

All brown rice can be used instead of an equal quantity of the long-grain variety, but this will give the dish a heavier texture, making it difficult to form the molds.

Variations
Try different nuts instead of cashews, or a combination of varieties.

Add wild rice to the brown rice.

For a traditional but more expensive Paella, replace the paprika with saffron.

Garnish sliced baby sweetcorn (blanched); diced red and green pepper (blanched); sprigs of fresh thyme

Protein – low
Fat – medium
Fiber – medium

Delhi Lasagne

¾ cup lentils
½ cup chopped onion
1 clove garlic, finely chopped
2 tsp garam masala (Indian seasoning)
1 tbsp polyunsaturated oil
1 cup vegetable stock
1 tsp coriander
salt and freshly ground pepper
8 oz lasagne verdi
3 oz low-fat Cheddar cheese, grated
toasted cooked lentils
Sauce
2 tbsp polyunsaturated margarine
2 tbsp flour
1 cup low-fat milk
salt and freshly ground pepper

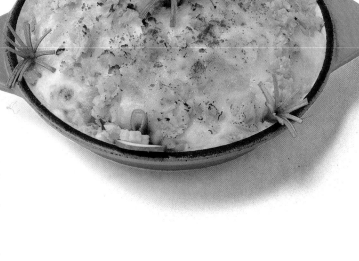

Soak the lentils as required (see page 4). Drain.

Sauté the onion, garlic and garam masala in the oil. Add the lentils and stir so that they are covered with the onion mixture. Mix in the stock. Bring to a boil and simmer gently, uncovered, for about 45 minutes, until the lentils are tender and the mixture thick. Stir in the coriander and season with salt and pepper.

Cook the lasagne in boiling, salted water until tender, then drain thoroughly. Meanwhile make the sauce. Melt the margarine, add the flour and make a roux (see page 103). Add the milk gradually and heat, stirring constantly, to make a smooth sauce. Allow to cook before stirring in the salt and pepper, and half the cheese.

In an ovenproof dish, layer the pasta, lentil mixture and sauce, finishing with a layer of the sauce. Sprinkle the top with the remaining grated cheese and toasted lentils. Bake at 400°F for 45–50 minutes, until golden brown.

Garnish slices of radish; baby sweetcorn; scallion fleuron (see page 99)

Protein – high
Fat – medium
Fiber – high

Lentil Roast

1 cup	lentils
4 oz	low-fat Cheddar cheese, grated
	1 onion, finely chopped
1 tsp	chopped fresh parsley
	pinch cayenne pepper
1 tbsp	lemon juice
	salt and freshly ground pepper
	1 medium egg
	chopped nuts

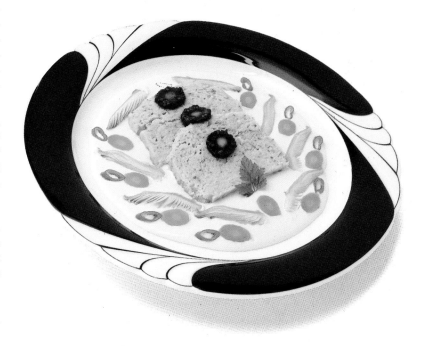

Soak the lentils as required (see page 4). Drain, place in a pot and cover with fresh cold water. Bring to a boil and boil rapidly for 10 minutes. Reduce the heat and simmer for 20–30 minutes. Check after 10 minutes, in case more water is needed. The mixture should cook to a stiff purée. Mix in the grated cheese, chopped onion, parsley, cayenne pepper and lemon juice. Season to taste.

Beat the egg lightly and mix into the lentil mixture. If the mixture is too moist, add some wholemeal breadcrumbs. Press the mixture into an oiled 1-lb loaf pan. Sprinkle lightly with chopped nuts. Bake at 375°F for 45–50 minutes, until the top is golden brown and the mixture feels firm to the touch.

Leave in the pan for 10 minutes before turning out. Serve with a sauce, such as mushroom (see page 96).

Variations
Divide the lentil mixture into three parts and layer with 1 cup sliced tomatoes.

Use yellow split peas instead of lentils.

Garnish oyster mushrooms; sliced carrot; scallion rings; sliced blackberry; fresh chervil

Protein – high
Fat – low
Fiber – medium

Soufflé Pancakes

Pancakes	
¹/₂ cup	*wholemeal flour*
	pinch salt
	1 egg, beaten
1 cup	*low-fat milk*
	polyunsaturated oil
Soufflé Filling	
2 tbsp	*polyunsaturated margarine*
2 tbsp	*flour*
¹/₂ cup	*low-fat milk*
	4 eggs
	salt and freshly ground pepper
2 oz	*low-fat Cheddar cheese, grated*
¹/₂ cup	*finely chopped walnuts*

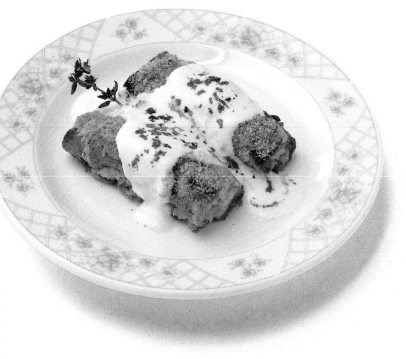

To make the pancakes, sift the flour and salt. Add the beaten egg and milk and blend to make a smooth batter. Make eight 6-inch pancakes.

To prepare the soufflé filling, melt the margarine, add the flour and cook for 3 minutes without allowing to darken in color. Blend in the milk gradually, stirring over a low heat until the sauce thickens and allow to cook. Let the mixture cool slightly and then add 2 whole eggs and 1 egg yolk (use remaining egg yolk in another recipe). Beat well and add seasoning and half the grated cheese. Turn the mixture into a bowl and stir in the walnuts. Whisk the remaining egg whites with a pinch of salt until stiff, add half to the soufflé mixture and mix well. Fold in the remaining egg white carefully.

Put about 2 tbsp of the soufflé filling across the center of each pancake and roll up carefully. Arrange in a well-oiled dish and sprinkle with the remaining cheese. Bake at 400°F for 15–20 minutes. Serve immediately.

Garnish yogurt and cream sauce; pinch of chopped fresh parsley; pinch of paprika; fresh thyme

Protein – high
Fat – high
Fiber – medium

Harvest Crumble

Crumble Topping
4 tbsp polyunsaturated margarine
1/2 cup wholemeal flour
2 tbsp rolled oats
2 oz low-fat Cheddar cheese, grated
2 tbsp walnuts, chopped
Filling
2 tbsp polyunsaturated margarine
3/4 cup diced celery
1/2 cup chopped red onions
1 cup sliced white cabbage
1 cup diced baby turnips
1/3 cup sliced baby sweetcorn
2 tbsp wholemeal flour
1/2 cup vegetable stock
3/4 cup canned tomatoes, chopped
1/2 cup low-fat milk
2 tsp chopped fresh parsley
salt and freshly ground pepper

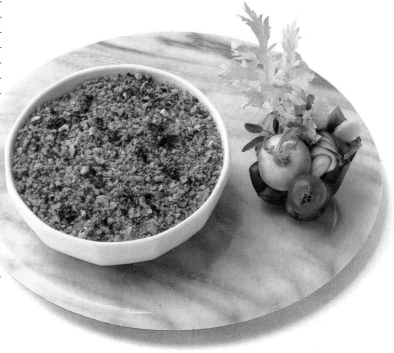

To make the crumble topping, rub the margarine into the flour and oats, then stir in the cheese and walnuts.

To make the filling, melt the margarine in a pan and sauté the celery, onion, cabbage, turnip and sweetcorn for 2 minutes, without allowing the vegetables to change color. Sprinkle with the flour, stir and cook for an additional 2 minutes. Gradually add the stock. Add the tomatoes, milk, parsley, salt and pepper, and bring to a boil, stirring constantly, until the sauce thickens. Allow to cook.

Put the filling into a dish and cover with the crumble topping. Bake at 375°F for 20 minutes, or until the crumble has browned.

Variation
Add crumbled blue cheese instead of Cheddar and replace the margarine with nut butter in the topping.

Garnish chopped parsley; green pepper filled with tomato, celery head, turnip, red onion and baby sweetcorn

Protein – medium
Fat – high
Fiber – high

Gumbo Stew

²/₃ cup	dried haricot beans
½ lb	okra
2 tbsp	polyunsaturated oil
	1 onion, chopped
	1 clove garlic, finely chopped
	1 green pepper, chopped
	1 green chilli, sliced
2 cups	canned tomatoes, chopped
¼ cup	tomato purée
	salt and freshly ground pepper
2 tsp	chopped fresh mixed herbs (thyme, chives, basil and oregano)
2 cups	vegetable stock, made with 1 stock cube
1 tsp	raw cane sugar
1 tsp	red wine vinegar

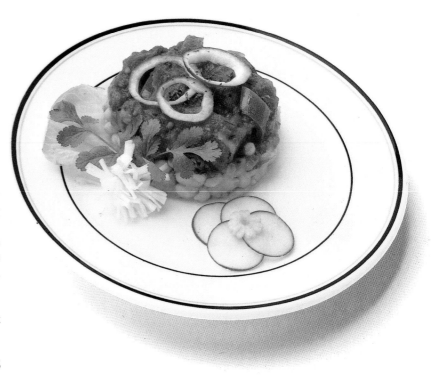

Soak the haricot beans overnight (see page 4). Drain, rinse and place in a pot of cold water. Bring to a boil and cook rapidly for 10 minutes. Reduce the heat and simmer for about 1½ hours. Drain. Alternatively use 2 cups canned or cooked haricot beans.

To prepare the okra, wash and dry, then cut off the stems without damaging or breaking open the pods.

Heat the oil in a pan and stir-fry the okra, onion and garlic for 5 minutes. Add the pepper, chilli, tomatoes, tomato purée, seasoning and herbs. Stir in the stock. Bring to a boil and simmer for 15 minutes. Stir in the sugar and vinegar. Simmer for an additional 5 minutes and serve.

Suggested Presentation
Using a small flan ring, make a base with the haricot beans. Top with the gumbo, remove the flan ring and garnish.

Garnish red onion rings; scallion fleuron (see page 99); radish; chicory; fresh oregano

Protein – medium
Fat – high
Fiber – high

Canneloni Verdi

12 canneloni verdi tubes or lasagne verdi sheets
2 tbsp polyunsaturated oil
½ cup chopped onions
1 clove garlic, finely chopped
2 cups sliced mushrooms
¾ lb zucchini, sliced
1 tsp fresh oregano, chopped
¾ cup canned tomatoes, chopped
1 tbsp tomato purée
salt and freshly ground pepper
1 oz Parmesan cheese, grated
Sauce
1 cup low-fat milk
1 onion clouté (see page 102)
2 tbsp polyunsaturated margarine
2 tbsp flour
2 oz Ricotta cheese

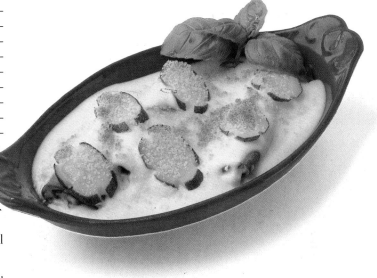

Cook the canneloni tubes or lasagne sheets in boiling water until tender. Drain and refresh in cold water.

Heat the oil and sauté the onion and garlic. Add the mushrooms and zucchini and sauté. Add the oregano, tomatoes, and tomato purée and sauté for 2–3 minutes. Add a little vegetable stock or water. Cover and cook gently for 10–15 minutes, then season to taste.

To make the sauce, heat the milk with the onion clouté. Melt the margarine in a pan, add the flour and make a roux (see page 103). Remove the onion and add the milk gradually. Heat, stirring constantly, until the sauce thickens. Allow to cook. Add the Ricotta cheese.

Spoon a little of the vegetable mixture into the canneloni tubes. Alternatively, spoon the mixture onto the lasagne sheets and roll up.

Arrange in a dish and cover generously with the sauce. Sprinkle with the Parmesan and bake at 350°F for 30 minutes.

Variation
Replace the vegetables with a sauce made from cooked beans and tomatoes.

Garnish canelled (see page 102) and sliced zucchini; fresh basil

Protein – high
Fat – high
Fiber – high

Harvest Pancakes

½ cup   plain wholemeal flour
pinch salt
pinch ground nutmeg
1 egg, beaten
1 cup   low-fat milk
polyunsaturated oil

To make the batter, sift the flour, salt and nutmeg. Add the beaten egg and milk and blend to make a smooth batter. Make eight 6-inch pancakes. Fill the pancakes with the chosen filling and serve immediately.

Suggested Fillings
Ratatouille and grated cheese (use ¼ cup cheese per serving)

Creamed spinach and Parmesan cheese, as shown in the photograph garnished with paprika and mint leaves (top the pancakes with Béchamel and yogurt cheese sauce, see page 96)

Cooked lentils and cashew nuts mixed with plain yogurt

Asparagus, mushrooms, leeks or broccoli in a sour cream or Béchamel sauce

Sweetcorn and red or green pepper in a mustard sauce (use 1 cup Béchamel sauce, see page 96, flavored with wholegrain mustard for 4 servings)

Crème fraîche with herbs (allow 6 tbsp low-fat crème fraîche per serving)

Stir-fried vegetables (fry some scallions, peas, beansprouts, mushrooms and walnuts; add a soy sauce thickened with a little cornflour)

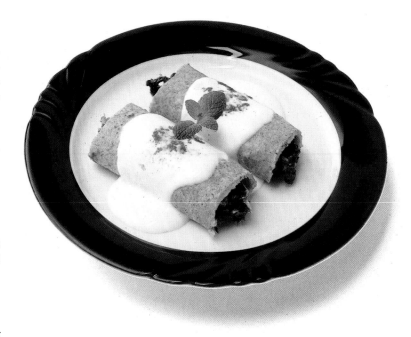

Variations
Use different flours and add such ingredients as chopped spinach, herbs and nuts to the batter mixture.

Fold the pancakes into envelopes; roll into cornets; stack to make a cake, layered with filling, and cut into wedges to serve.

Garnish plain yogurt; fresh mint; pinch of paprika

Analysis for Pancake only

Protein – low
Fat – medium
Fiber – low

Baked Broccoli with Tomato

2½ cups	broccoli florets
4 tbsp	polyunsaturated margarine
½ cup	finely chopped onions
1 clove garlic, finely chopped	
1¼ cups	sliced mushrooms
¼ cup	wholemeal flour
2 tbsp	tomato purée
1½ cups	vegetable stock
½ cup	canned tomatoes, chopped
salt and freshly ground pepper	
2 oz	low-fat Cheddar cheese, grated
2 oz	Mozzarella cheese, diced

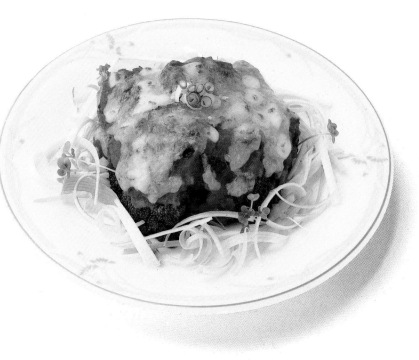

Cook the broccoli in boiling water until just tender. Drain and place in an ovenproof dish.

Melt the margarine and cook the onion, just until soft. Add the garlic and mushrooms and cook for 2 minutes. Stir in the flour and cook for 5 minutes, stirring constantly. Add the tomato purée. Stir in the stock and bring to a boil. Add the tomatoes, salt and pepper. Return to a boil and adjust the seasoning.

Pour the tomato sauce evenly over the broccoli. Mix the Cheddar and Mozzarella together and sprinkle on top. Bake at 350°F for 30 minutes. Serve with hash brown potatoes.

Variation
Top with a nutty crumble mixture.

Garnish scallion and cucumber shavings;
mustard and cress

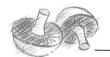

Protein – medium
Fat – medium
Fiber – medium

Singapore Stroganoff

1 tbsp	polyunsaturated oil
¹/₂ cup	sliced onions
¹/₂ cup	mixed peppers, cut in strips
¹/₂ cup	carrots, cut in thin strips
¹/₄ lb	zucchini, cut in thin strips
¹/₂ cup	sliced water chestnuts
1 tsp	fresh thyme, chopped
	salt and freshly ground pepper
¹/₄ cup	mixed chopped nuts, toasted
	chopped fresh parsley
8 oz	wholewheat spaghetti, cooked

Sauce

2 tbsp	polyunsaturated margarine
1¹/₄ cups	sliced mushrooms
2 tbsp	flour
1 cup	low-fat milk
3 oz	low-fat soft cheese
	pinch ground nutmeg
	salt and freshly ground pepper
¹/₄ cup	plain yogurt

To make the sauce, melt the margarine and sauté the mushrooms. Add the flour to make a roux (see page 103). Gradually add the milk and heat, stirring, to make a smooth sauce. Allow to cook. Stir in the soft cheese and season well. Just before serving, stir in the yogurt.

Reserve some vegetables for garnish and blanch in boiling water for 30 seconds.

Heat the oil and sauté the onion. Add the peppers, carrots, zucchini, water chestnuts and thyme and sauté without allowing them to change color. Season with salt and pepper. Put the mixture in an earthenware dish. Cover with the sauce, arrange blanched vegetables and top with the mixed nuts and parsley.

Serve with wholewheat spaghetti or noodles, or brown rice.

Garnish scallion fleuron (see page 99); radicchio; fresh chervil; curly endive; sliced mushrooms

Protein – medium
Fat – medium
Fiber – high

Italian-style Peppers

4 large whole peppers (red, yellow or green)
Filling
1¼ cups sliced mushrooms
¾ cup brown rice, cooked
2 tsp chopped fresh parsley
1 tsp chopped mixed fresh herbs (thyme, basil, chives and oregano)
⅓ cup fresh or frozen peas
1 cup coarsely chopped mixed nuts
salt and freshly ground pepper
2 tbsp polyunsaturated margarine
2 tbsp wholemeal flour
1 cup low-fat milk
¼ cup plain yogurt
2 oz Mozzarella cheese, sliced

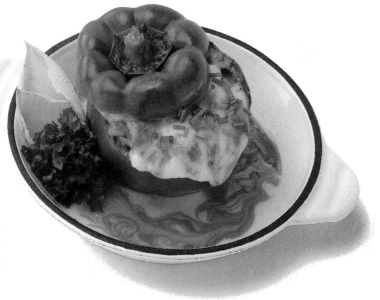

Prepare the peppers (see page 5).

To make the filling, cook the mushrooms gently in their own juices. Stir in the rice, parsley, mixed herbs, peas and nuts. Season well. Melt the margarine in another pan, add the flour and make a roux (see page 103). Add the milk gradually, stirring over a low heat until the sauce thickens. Allow to cook, then add the yogurt, taking care that the sauce does not boil. Combine the rice mixture with the sauce and fill the peppers. Top with the Mozzarella slices. Replace the pepper lids.

Arrange the peppers in a greased ovenproof dish. Bake at 400°F for about 40 minutes, until tender. Cover with greased paper for the first 20 minutes. Serve with a coulis of Béchamel sauce (see page 96) and lace with tomato sauce (see page 96) (using a fork to twirl sauces lightly) as shown in the photograph.

Variation
Replace the rice with cooked bulgur wheat (see page 102).

Garnish chicory; red leaf lettuce; snipped fresh chives

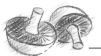

Protein – medium
Fat – high
Fiber – medium

Chickpeas Provençale

⅓ cup   dried chickpeas
2 tbsp   polyunsaturated oil
1¼ cups   diced onions
2 large eggplants, cut into cubes
½ cup   yellow peppers, cut into strips
½ cup   red peppers, cut into strips
½ lb   zucchini, sliced
1 clove garlic, finely chopped
2 cups   canned tomatoes, chopped
2 tbsp   tomato purée
1 cup   vegetable stock
1 fresh bay leaf
2 tsp   chopped mixed fresh herbs (thyme, basil, chives and oregano)
salt and freshly ground pepper
1 lb   fresh noodles, mixed spinach and egg, cooked
or
½ lb   dried noodles, cooked

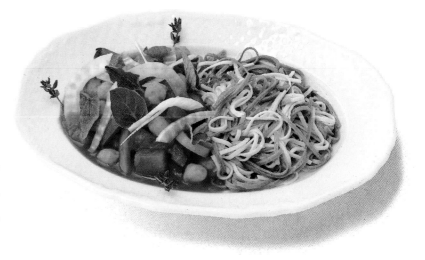

Soak the chickpeas overnight (see page 4). Drain, rinse and place in a pot of cold water. Bring to a boil and cook rapidly for 10 minutes. Reduce the heat and simmer for 1–1½ hours. Drain. Alternatively use 1 cup canned or cooked chickpeas.

Heat the oil and sauté the onion until tender. Add the eggplant, peppers, zucchini and garlic and continue to cook, covered, until the vegetables are soft. Stir in the tomatoes, tomato purée, stock and chickpeas. Add the bay leaf and mixed herbs. Season with salt and pepper and simmer, uncovered, for 20–30 minutes.

Serve with noodles.

Variations
Stuff green peppers with the mixture and bake until the peppers are tender.

Replace the noodles with brown rice.

Garnish thin slices of fennel; fresh oregano; fresh thyme

Protein – high
Fat – medium
Fiber – high

Vegetable Cheesecake

Base
6 tbsp   polyunsaturated margarine
¹⁄₃ cup   wholemeal breadcrumbs, toasted
¹⁄₄ cup   oatmeal
pinch ground nutmeg
Topping
¹⁄₂ cup   finely chopped onions
1 clove garlic, finely chopped
1 tbsp   polyunsaturated oil
¹⁄₂ cup   finely sliced zucchini
¹⁄₂ cup   finely sliced carrots
1 tsp   finely chopped fresh basil or rosemary
1 tsp   finely chopped fresh parsley
salt and freshly ground pepper
1 cup   cottage cheese
1 oz   Parmesan cheese
2 eggs

Melt the margarine and add the breadcrumbs, oatmeal and nutmeg. Press the breadcrumb mixture into the base of an oiled flan dish.

Sauté the onion and garlic in the oil until softened. Add the vegetables and herbs and cook gently until tender. Season with salt and pepper. Meanwhile, beat together the cheeses and eggs. Combine with the vegetables. Turn the mixture into the flan dish and bake at 375°F for about 20 minutes, until set. Serve hot or cold.

Variations
Vary the vegetable content or try different herbs.

Serve a spicy tomato sauce (see page 97) as an accompaniment.

Use tofu instead of the cottage cheese.

Garnish cherry tomato flower; fresh basil leaves; pink grapefruit slices; raspberries

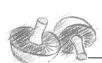

Protein – high
Fat – high
Fiber – medium

Suppli

2 tbsp   polyunsaturated margarine
½ cup   chopped onion
1½ cups   long-grain rice
¼ cup   dry white wine
4 cups   vegetable stock
½ tsp   saffron
salt and freshly ground pepper
3 eggs
1 oz   Parmesan cheese, grated
2 tbsp   low-fat milk
4 oz   Mozzarella cheese, cut in ½-inch cubes
2 tbsp   flour
¼ cup   wholemeal breadcrumbs
polyunsaturated oil

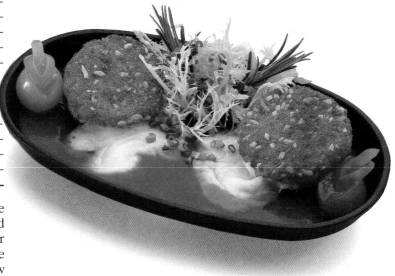

Melt the margarine and sauté the onion until tender. Add the rice and stir until the grains are coated. Add the wine, half the stock, and the saffron, salt and pepper. Bring to a boil, stirring well, and simmer until the liquid has evaporated. Add the remaining stock. Reduce the heat and cook, uncovered, until the liquid has been absorbed. Allow to cool.

Beat 2 of the eggs lightly with the Parmesan cheese and combine with the rice mixture. Beat the remaining egg with the milk for the egg wash. Mold the rice mixture into small cakes or balls. Put a cube of cheese in the center of each. Dip first in the flour, then the egg wash and coat with the breadcrumbs.

Fry in hot oil until golden brown. Drain and serve with a spicy sauce (see page 98).

Variation
Add different fresh herbs to the rice mixture, such as parsley, dill, thyme or tarragon.

Garnish feathered cherry tomato; curly endive; fresh rosemary; chopped scallion tops; chopped nuts

Protein – high
Fat – medium
Fiber – medium

Lentil and Cauliflower Spice

1 cup   lentils
2 tbsp   polyunsaturated oil
½ cup   finely chopped onion
1 tsp   ground turmeric
few drops chilli sauce
1 tsp   ground cumin
1 tsp   ground coriander
½ lime
1 head cauliflower
1½ cups   vegetable stock
2 tbsp   shredded coconut
2 tsp   potato flour (fecule)
2 tbsp   cold water
½ cup   cashew nuts
salt and freshly ground pepper

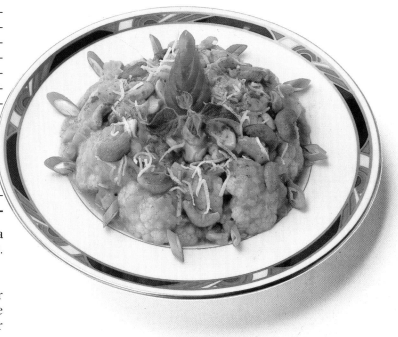

Soak the lentils as required (see page 4). Drain, rinse and place in a pot of cold water. Bring to a boil and cook rapidly for 10 minutes. Drain.

Heat the oil and sauté the onion. As it softens, add the spices. Stir well and cook for 30 seconds. Add the lentils and stir well to ensure each grain is coated. Squeeze in the lime juice. Break the cauliflower into florets and add, with the vegetable stock and coconut. Bring to a boil and simmer for 20 minutes. If a thicker sauce is required, mix the potato flour with the cold water to form a paste and stir in. Add the cashew nuts and simmer until the cauliflower is just cooked. Correct the seasoning with salt and pepper.

Serve on a bed of saffron rice or with naan bread. Wedges of lime would make a refreshing accompaniment.

Garnish sliced scallion tops; pinch of paprika; shredded coconut; toasted cashews; feathered cherry tomato; sprig of fresh oregano

Protein – high
Fat – high
Fiber – high

Lentil Duchesse

1 cup   lentils
4 tbsp   polyunsaturated margarine
1 onion, chopped
1 clove garlic, finely chopped
1 stalk celery, chopped
½ cup   carrots, grated
1¼ cups   sliced mushrooms
½ tsp   fresh thyme, chopped
½ tsp   fresh marjoram, chopped
1 tsp   tomato purée
salt and freshly ground pepper
vegetable stock
1½ lb   whipped potatoes

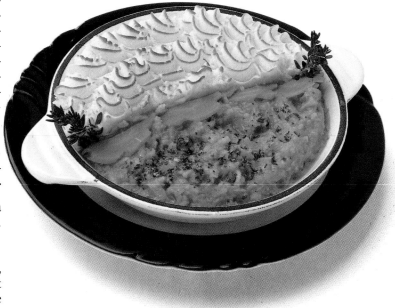

Soak the lentils as required (see page 4). Drain, rinse and place in a pot of cold water. Bring to a boil and cook rapidly for 10 minutes. Reduce the heat and simmer for 20–30 minutes. Drain.

Melt the margarine and sauté the vegetables for about 10 minutes, just until tender. Then add the lentils, herbs, tomato purée and salt and pepper, mixing thoroughly. Add a little vegetable stock if the mixture appears dry.

Spoon the lentil mixture into an oiled, shallow, ovenproof dish or individual dishes. Spread or pipe the whipped potatoes on top and bake at 400°F for 30–40 minutes, until golden-brown.

Variations
Serve with a tomato or mushroom sauce (see page 96).

Add chopped nuts to the potatoes to vary the texture.

Replace the lentils with cooked beans, such as aduki beans or black-eyed peas.

Garnish sliced carrot; fresh thyme; chopped fresh parsley

Protein – high
Fat – medium
Fiber – high

Wild Green Risotto

4 cups   broccoli florets
½ cup   sliced onions
1 clove garlic, finely chopped
1 tbsp   polyunsaturated margarine
2 tsp   chopped mixed fresh herbs (oregano, thyme, basil and chives)
salt and freshly ground pepper
4 tbsp   polyunsaturated margarine
¼ cup   wholemeal flour
2 tbsp   tomato purée
2 cups   low-fat milk
½ cup   brown rice
2 tbsp   wild rice
1 tbsp   pine nuts
pinch chopped fresh basil

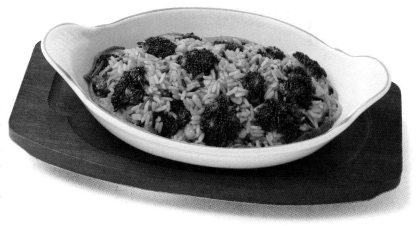

Reserve a few broccoli florets for garnish. Place the remainder in a large pot with a little water, the onion, garlic, 1 tbsp polyunsaturated margarine, herbs and seasoning. Bring to a boil, reduce the heat, cover and cook the vegetables until tender but still crisp. Place in a greased ovenproof dish.

Make the sauce by melting the margarine, adding the flour and cooking for 1–2 minutes over a low heat. Add the tomato purée and gradually add the milk. Heat, stirring constantly, until the sauce thickens. Season and allow to cook.

Cook both rices according to the instructions on the packets. Drain and mix with the pine nuts and basil. Combine with the sauce and pour over broccoli. Bake at 350°F for 15 minutes.

Variations
Use spring greens or purple sprouting broccoli instead of green broccoli.

Substitute sunflower seeds for the pine nuts, adding a little grated Parmesan cheese.

Mix toasted, flaked almonds with the rice.

Garnish cooked broccoli florets

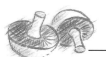

Protein – medium
Fat – medium
Fiber – high

Wholesome Hotpot

²/₃ cup	dried butter beans
1 cup	chopped onions
1 cup	chopped celery
1 cup	sliced carrots
¹/₃ cup	sliced leeks
1 cup	vegetable stock
	salt and freshly ground pepper
¹/₂ lb	potatoes, thinly sliced
2 tbsp	polyunsaturated margarine, melted

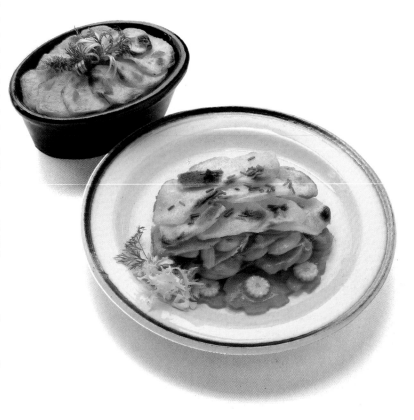

Soak the butter beans overnight (see page 3). Drain, rinse and place in a pot of cold water. Bring to a boil and cook rapidly for 10 minutes. Reduce heat and simmer for about 1 hour. Drain. Alternatively use 2 cups canned or cooked butter beans.

Mix the beans with the onion, celery, carrot, leek, stock, salt and pepper. Spoon into individual serving dishes. Arrange the sliced potatoes on top and brush with the melted margarine. Bake at 350°F for 45–60 minutes.

Variations
To make a more substantial dish, add 2 tbsp wholegrain barley with the vegetables and stock.

Sprinkle with sesame seeds before putting in the oven to give a more unusual flavor.

Garnish scallion fleuron (see page 99) and fresh dill; or endive, fresh dill, chopped fresh chives and sliced baby sweetcorn

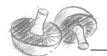

Protein – low
Fat – low
Fiber – high

Eggplant and Zucchini Bake

½ lb	eggplant, sliced
3 tbsp	polyunsaturated oil
	flour for dusting
½ cup	chopped onion
1 cup	canned tomatoes, chopped
	2 eggs
4 oz	cottage cheese
½ cup	plain yogurt
½ lb	zucchini, sliced thin
	salt and freshly ground pepper
1 oz	Parmesan cheese, grated

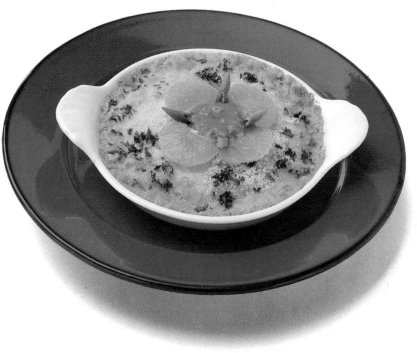

Sprinkle the eggplant slices with salt and allow to drain. Dry with paper toweling.

Heat the oil. Dust the eggplant with flour and sauté until golden and soft. Remove from the pan. Sauté the onion until soft. Add the tomatoes and simmer until the mixture reduces to a pulp. Let cool.

Beat the eggs with the cottage cheese and yogurt. Combine with the cooled tomato mixture. Add seasoning. Put a layer of eggplant and zucchini in a greased ovenproof dish and cover with some of the tomato mixture. Sprinkle with some of the Parmesan cheese. Continue in layers, finishing with a topping of cheese. Bake at 375°F for 40 minutes, or until golden.

Variation
For a more expensive alternative, try Ricotta cheese instead of cottage cheese.

Garnish tomato sauce (see page 96); segments of clementine orange; fresh chives; chopped fresh parsley

Protein – medium
Fat – high
Fiber – low

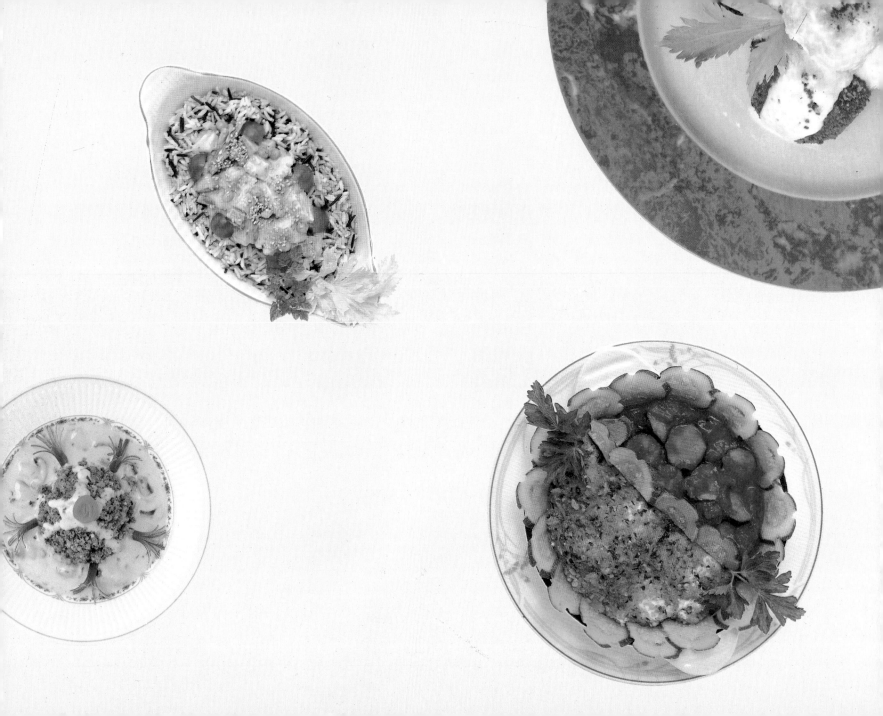

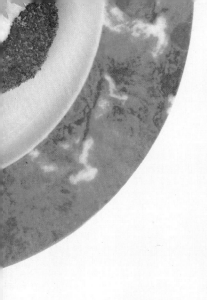
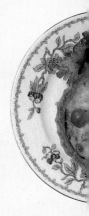
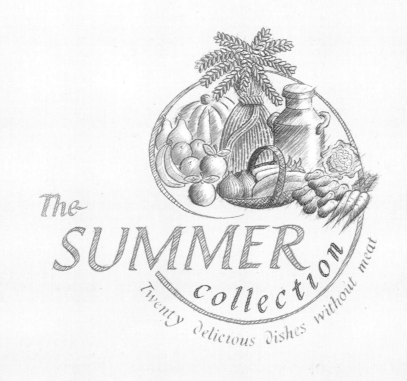

The

SUMMER
collection

Twenty delicious dishes without meat

"Hot" Peppers

¾ cup   bulgur wheat
4 yellow peppers
2 tbsp   polyunsaturated oil
½ cup   chopped onions
2 tsp   chilli seasoning
¾ cup   canned tomatoes, chopped
2 tbsp   tomato purée
1 tsp   ground cumin
½ vegetable stock cube, crumbled
salt and freshly ground pepper
1 cup   plain yogurt
½ cup   finely chopped cucumber

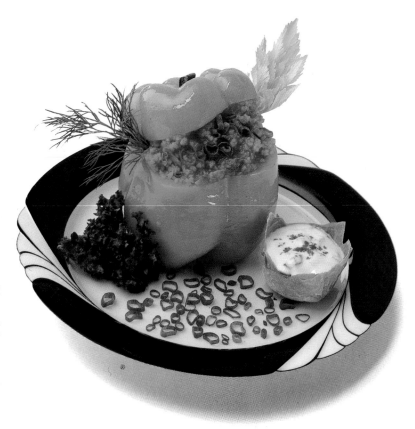

Cover the bulgur wheat with twice its volume of cold water and soak for 20 minutes. Drain well. Meanwhile prepare the peppers (see page 5).

Heat the oil and sauté the onion with the chilli seasoning for 3–4 minutes. Add the tomatoes, tomato purée, cumin, crumbled stock cube, a little water and drained bulgur wheat. Cook, stirring, for 1–2 minutes. Add seasoning. Fill the peppers with the chilli mixture and replace the pepper lids. Cover with greased foil and bake at 375°F for about 40 minutes.

Heat the yogurt gently with the cucumber. Whisk lightly, season and serve hot or cold as an accompaniment to the peppers.

Variation
Add finely diced vegetables such as mushrooms, zucchini or eggplant to the bulgur wheat.

Garnish red leaf lettuce; celery top; fresh dill; snipped fresh chives; yogurt and cucumber dressing in a filo pastry basket (see page 5)

Protein – low
Fat – medium
Fiber – medium

Mushroom Crunch

Crunch

4 tbsp	polyunsaturated margarine
1/2 cup	fresh wholemeal breadcrumbs
3 oz	low-fat Cheddar cheese, grated
3/4 cup	chopped mixed nuts
1 tsp	chopped fresh mixed herbs
1 clove garlic, finely chopped	

Sauce

4 tbsp	polyunsaturated margarine
1 1/4 cups	sliced mushrooms
1/4 cup	flour
2 cups	low-fat milk
salt and freshly ground pepper	
1 tsp	chopped fresh mixed herbs (oregano, chives, basil and chervil)

To make the crunch, rub the margarine into the breadcrumbs, add the remaining ingredients and mix well. Shape into individual mounds and bake at 425°F for 15 minutes.

Meanwhile, melt the margarine for the sauce and sauté the mushrooms for a few minutes. Remove the mushrooms and reserve. Add the flour to the remaining liquid to make a roux (see page 103), and gradually add the milk. Heat, stirring constantly, until the sauce thickens, and allow to cook. Add the mushrooms, seasoning and mixed herbs. Spoon some of the sauce over each serving plate, place a crunch mound on each and coat with the remaining sauce.

Variation
Replace the mushrooms with other vegetables such as leeks, celery or asparagus.

Garnish yellow cherry tomato rose;
scallion fleurons (see page 99)

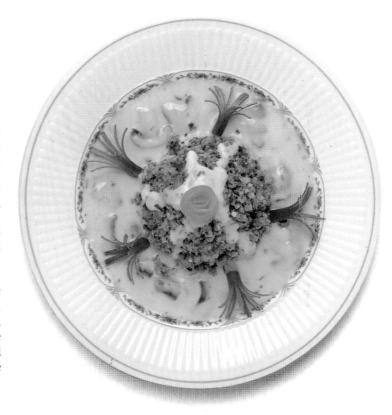

Protein – high
Fat – high
Fiber – medium

Ratatouille

1 tbsp	*polyunsaturated oil*
1¼ cups	*finely chopped onions*
2 cloves garlic, finely chopped	
½ lb	*zucchini, cut into 1 × 1½-inch dice*
½ lb	*chayote squash, peeled and cut into 1 × 1½-inch dice*
1 lb	*fresh tomatoes, skinned and chopped, or canned tomatoes, chopped*
2 red peppers, roughly chopped	
1 tsp	*chopped fresh parsley*
1 vegetable stock cube, crumbled	
1 tsp	*chopped fresh basil*
salt and freshly ground pepper	

Heat the oil and sauté the onion and garlic until soft. Add all the remaining ingredients, cover and simmer for 30 minutes.

Serve with wholewheat pasta, brown rice or potatoes or as a side dish to accompany a flan or savory casserole.

Variations
Use as a base for other dishes, such as ratatouille crumble, or as a filling for savory pancakes.

Add cooked chickpeas or lentils to increase the protein content.

Garnish blanched, finely diced green and red peppers; chopped fresh parsley

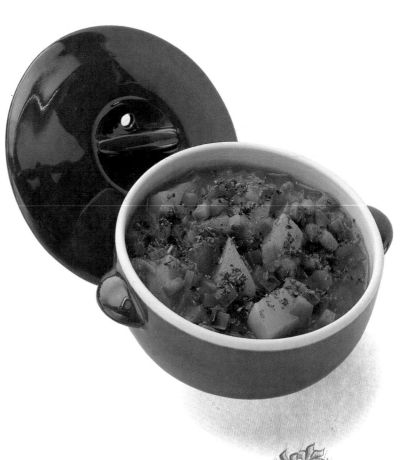

Protein – low
Fat – low
Fiber – low

Croquettes Mont Blanc

1 lb	parsnips, rutabagas, or other root vegetables, diced
1 cup	low-fat milk
1/3 cup	finely chopped onions
2 tbsp	polyunsaturated margarine
1 tsp	chopped fresh chives
1 egg, beaten	
1/2 cup	finely chopped chestnuts
1/4 cup	wholemeal flour
salt and freshly ground pepper	
Coating	
1 egg	
2 tbsp	low-fat milk
1/2 cup	fresh breadcrumbs
polyunsaturated oil	
Sauce	
2 tbsp	polyunsaturated margarine
2 tbsp	flour
1 cup	low-fat milk
3 oz	low-fat soft cheese

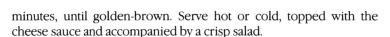

Put the parsnips in a pot with the milk, bring to a boil and simmer, uncovered, until tender and most of the liquid has been absorbed. Drain off any excess liquid, then mash. Sauté the onion in the margarine until soft. Add the onion, chives, egg, chestnuts and flour to the parsnip mixture. Season well and chill until firm.

To make the sauce, melt the margarine, add the flour and cook gently for 1–2 minutes. Gradually add the milk and heat, stirring constantly, until the sauce thickens. Allow to cook before stirring in the cheese.

Lightly whisk the egg and milk for the coating. Just before serving, shape the parsnip mixture into balls. Dip each into the egg wash and roll in breadcrumbs. Deep- or shallow-fry the croquettes for about 5 minutes, until golden-brown. Serve hot or cold, topped with the cheese sauce and accompanied by a crisp salad.

Variation

A red wine or cranberry sauce would make a suitable alternative to the cheese sauce.

Garnish grated Parmesan cheese; paprika; celery tops

Protein – high
Fat – medium
Fiber – high

Lima Bean Curry

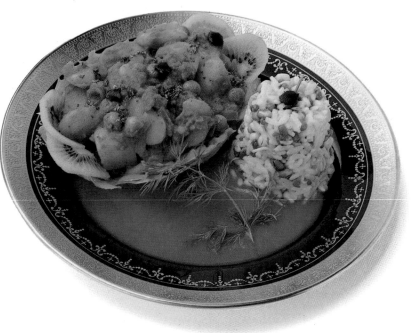

¾ cup   dried butter beans
1 tbsp   polyunsaturated oil
½ cup   chopped onions
1 clove garlic, finely chopped
1 tsp   curry powder
1 tsp   paprika
1 cup   canned tomatoes, roughly chopped
1 lb   potatoes, peeled and cubed
2 fresh bay leaves
1½ cups   vegetable stock
½ cup   peas, fresh or frozen
salt and freshly ground pepper

Soak the butter beans overnight (see page 3). Drain, rinse and place in a pot of cold water. Bring to a boil and cook rapidly for 10 minutes. Reduce heat and simmer for 1–1½ hours. Drain. Alternatively use 2 cups canned or cooked beans.

Heat the oil and sauté the onion and garlic for 5 minutes; do not allow to turn brown. Stir in the spices and cook for a few minutes before adding the tomatoes. Cover and simmer for an additional 5 minutes, then add the potatoes and bay leaves. Add the stock and stir well. Simmer gently until the potatoes are nearly cooked, add the butter beans, peas and seasoning and cook for an additional 5–6 minutes.

Serve accompanied by mixed brown and white rice, combined with beansprouts (one part to four parts rice), pressed into a dariole mold (see page 102) and turned out onto a tomato sauce base.

Variation
Add ⅓ cup raisins or sultanas and 1 tbsp apricot jam to give the curry a slightly sweet taste.

Garnish sliced kiwi fruit; chopped fresh parsley; thinly sliced black olive; sprig of dill

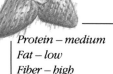

Protein – medium
Fat – low
Fiber – high

Capsicum and Chickpea Couscous

⅓ cup   dried chickpeas
1 cup   couscous
2 tbsp   polyunsaturated oil
½ cup   chopped onions
1 eggplant, diced
1 red pepper, diced
1 green pepper, diced
2 carrots, sliced
½ tsp   ground cumin
½ tsp   ground coriander
½ tsp   turmeric
1 cup   canned tomatoes, chopped
1 tbsp   tomato purée
1 cup   vegetable stock
2 zucchini, sliced
⅓ cup   sultanas or raisins
salt and freshly ground pepper
2 tsp   chopped fresh parsley

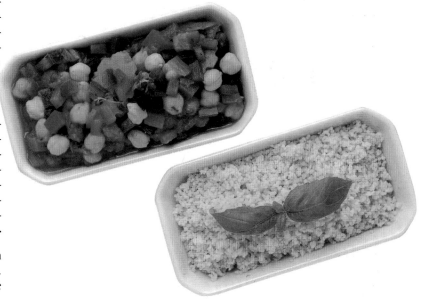

Soak the chickpeas overnight (see page 4). Drain, rinse, and place in a pot of cold water. Bring to a boil and cook rapidly for 10 minutes. Reduce heat and simmer for 1–1½ hours. Drain. Alternatively use 1 cup canned or cooked chickpeas.

Soak the couscous in cold water for 15 minutes, and drain. Heat the oil, add the onion, eggplant, peppers and carrot and sauté for 5 minutes, stirring frequently. Stir in the cumin, coriander, turmeric, tomatoes, tomato purée and stock. Bring to a boil and stir well. Cover and simmer for 20 minutes. Add the chickpeas, zucchini, sultanas and seasoning. Stir well. Cover and simmer for an additional 20 minutes. Cook couscous according to instructions on the packet.

Spread the couscous over a serving dish and fluff with a fork. Add the parsley to the vegetable mixture and serve with the couscous.

Variation
Other grains, such as bulgur wheat, can be substituted for the couscous.

Garnish diced peppers, blanched; fresh thyme; fresh basil (on couscous)

Protein – low
Fat – medium
Fiber – medium

Chayote Almondine

1 medium chayote squash, seeded, peeled and thickly sliced
2 onions, chopped
2 tbsp   polyunsaturated oil
1 red pepper, chopped
1¼ cups   sliced mushrooms
½ cup   ground almonds
½ cup   wholemeal breadcrumbs
2 eggs, beaten together with ½ cup water
1 tsp   chopped fresh mixed herbs (oregano, chives, basil and chervil)
2 tbsp   skimmed milk powder
salt and freshly ground pepper
2 tbsp   tomato purée
2 tomatoes, sliced
4 oz   Mozzarella cheese
¼ cup   almonds

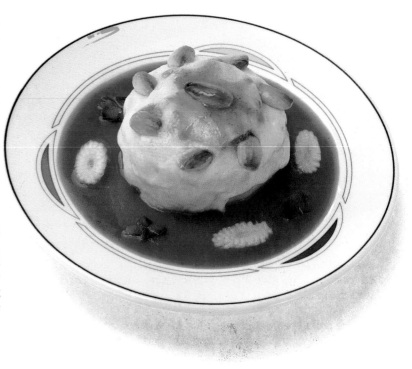

Boil the chayote slices for 5 minutes and refresh with cold water.

Sauté the onions in the oil. Add the red pepper and mushrooms and sauté for 1–2 minutes. Mix with the ground almonds, breadcrumbs, eggs, herbs, skimmed milk powder and seasoning to obtain a moist mixture. Spread the chayote slices with tomato purée and pile on the filling. Top with sliced tomatoes, Mozzarella cheese and a sprinkling of almonds. Bake at 350°F for 30 minutes and serve with barbecue sauce (see page 98).

Variation
Replace the eggs with almond butter.

Garnish toasted almonds; sliced baby sweetcorn; finely chopped green pepper

Protein – high
Fat – high
Fiber – high

Garbanzo Fritters

¾ cup   dried chickpeas
1 small onion, quartered
2 cloves garlic, finely chopped
4 slices (4 oz)   wholemeal bread
½ tsp   cumin seeds
3 small red chillies, crushed
1 egg, beaten
2 tsp   chopped fresh parsley
salt and freshly ground pepper
¼ cup   wholemeal breadcrumbs
vegetable oil
4 wholemeal pita breads, warmed
endive, onion and tomato slices

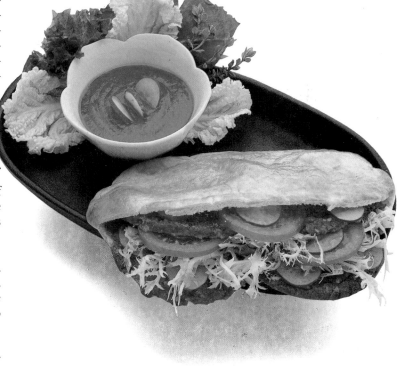

Soak chickpeas overnight (see page 4). Drain, rinse, place in a pot of cold water, bring to a boil and cook rapidly for 10 minutes. Reduce heat and simmer for 1–1½ hours. Drain. Alternatively use 2½ cups canned or cooked chickpeas.

Place chickpeas, onion, garlic, bread, cumin seeds and chillies in a food processor or blender. Process until smooth and turn into a bowl. Add egg, parsley and seasoning and mix well. Form the mixture into eight balls. Coat each ball in breadcrumbs and flatten to give an oval shape.

Half-fill a deep-fryer or deep saucepan with oil. Heat to 375°F and fry the chickpea fritters for about 3 minutes. Drain well. Cut each pita bread in half, cut a fritter in half and place inside the pita with a little endive and a few slices of onion and tomato. Serve hot, with barbecue sauce (see page 98).

Variation
Serve with a refreshing relish, a lemon-flavored mayonnaise or a yogurt dressing.

Garnish red leaf lettuce; Chinese cabbage; radicchio; fresh thyme

Protein – high
Fat – low
Fiber – high

Nutty Burgers

½ cup	chopped onions
1 tbsp	polyunsaturated oil
1 cup	finely chopped mixed nuts
1 cup	finely chopped peanuts
2 tbsp	peanut butter
⅔ cup	wholemeal breadcrumbs
1 tsp	chopped fresh mixed herbs (thyme, basil, oregano and chives)
1 tsp	chopped fresh parsley
	salt and freshly ground pepper
	vegetable stock

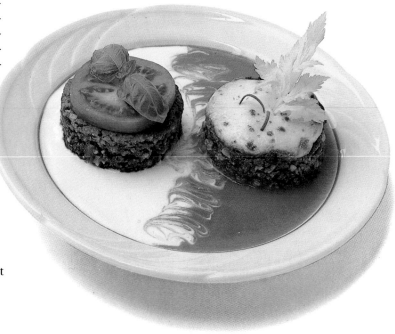

Sauté the onion in the oil, then stir in the mixed nuts, peanuts, peanut butter, breadcrumbs, herbs, parsley and seasoning. Mix well, adding sufficient stock to bind. Shape the mixture into burgers. Put on an oiled pan and bake at 400°F for 30 minutes, turning once.

Serve with a tomato slice or corn relish, or a hot tomato sauce.

Variation
Add other vegetables or different nuts to enhance this basic nut burger recipe.

Garnish half tomato sauce (see page 96), half cheese sauce (see page 96) on serving plate; 1 burger topped with tomato and fresh oregano; 1 burger topped with melted Mozzarella; celery top

Protein – medium
Fat – high
Fiber – medium

Omelette Collection

Omelette (serves 1)
3 eggs
salt and freshly ground pepper
cold water
1 tbsp   polyunsaturated margarine

Whisk the eggs with seasoning and a dash of water. Melt the margarine in an omelette pan. When it begins to foam, pour in the egg and as it sets, break up lightly with a fork, ensuring all the mixture is cooked. Add the chosen filling and when the bottom is lightly browned, fold and tip onto a serving dish.

Suggestions for Fillings

Spinach omelette: chopped spinach, mixed with small cubes of Mozzarella cheese (as shown in the photograph), served with a tomato sauce (see page 96), garnished with feathered cherry tomato (see page 99), parsley, red chicory, Chinese cabbage, rosemary and thyme.

Nutty mushroom omelette: sliced mushrooms, sautéed with mixed chopped nuts and a little yeast extract.

Pasta omelette: mix cooked wholewheat pasta into the egg mixture prior to cooking. Pour into the pan and cook as for the basic omelette. Sprinkle Parmesan cheese in the center before turning out.

Spanish omelette: sauté chopped onions with diced green and red peppers. Add the egg mixture and cook without breaking up. When just set, turn the omelette over until the bottom is lightly browned. Do not fold.

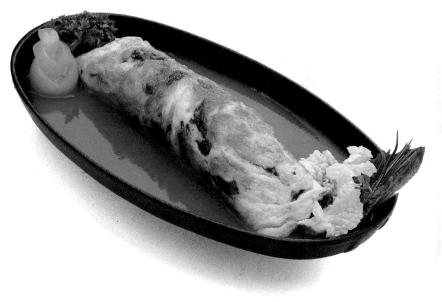

Analysis for Omelette only:

Protein – low
Fat – medium
Fiber – low

Cheddar Roast

2 tbsp	polyunsaturated margarine
½ cup	chopped onions
½ cup	grated carrots
1 cup	chopped mixed nuts
4 slices (4 oz)	wholemeal bread
1 cup	vegetable stock
1 tsp	yeast extract
2 tsp	chopped fresh mixed herbs (oregano, chives, thyme and basil)
	few drops Worcestershire sauce
	salt and freshly ground pepper
	2 tomatoes, sliced
2 oz	low-fat Cheddar cheese, grated

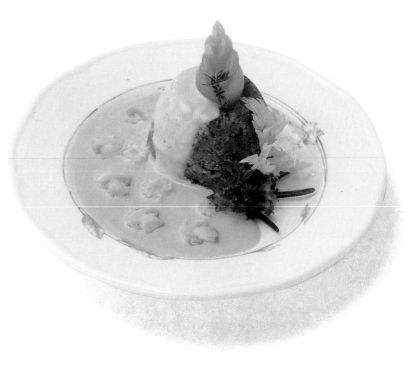

Melt the margarine and sauté the onions; add the carrots and continue to sauté. Remove from the heat. Grind the nuts and bread together. Heat the vegetable stock with the yeast extract together until just boiling. Combine all the ingredients except the tomatoes and cheese and gradually add sufficient stock to obtain a firm mixture. Half-fill four small pudding molds or a loaf pan with the mixture and cover with a layer of sliced tomato and grated cheese, then fill with the remaining mixture. Bake at 350°F for 30 minutes, or until golden-brown.

Turn out and serve with a mushroom sauce (see page 96).

Variation

Omit the cheese and tomato to make a basic nut roast which can be served hot or cold or used as a filling for sandwiches and baked potatoes.

Garnish sliced mushrooms; sliced baby sweetcorn; feathered cherry tomato (see page 99); celery top; red leaf lettuce; rosemary and thyme

Protein – medium
Fat – high
Fiber – medium

Gardener's Delight

½ lb	wholemeal shortcrust pastry
2 tbsp	polyunsaturated margarine
2 tbsp	flour
1 cup	low-fat milk
4 oz	low-fat Cheddar cheese, grated
	salt and freshly ground pepper
½ cup	grated carrots
½ cup	thinly sliced leeks
½ cup	peas, fresh or frozen
½ cup	sweetcorn kernels

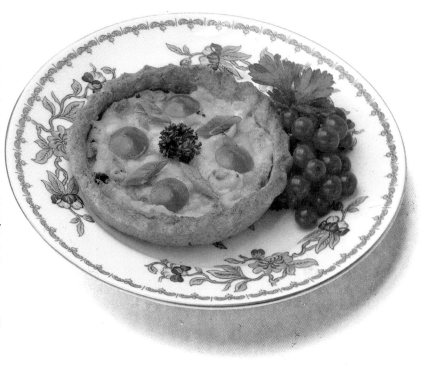

Line one large or four individual flan rings with the pastry and bake blind (see page 102).

To prepare the sauce, melt the margarine, add the flour and cook gently for 1–2 minutes. Gradually stir in the milk and heat, stirring constantly, until the sauce thickens. Allow to cook before adding half the cheese. Season. Combine the cheese sauce with all the vegetables. Divide the mixture evenly between the flans. Sprinkle with the remaining grated cheese and bake at 375°F for 30 minutes.

Variations
Use different flours, buckwheat for example, to make a more unusual pastry.

Vary the texture by adding nuts or oatmeal to the pastry.

Garnish sliced cherry tomato; sliced scallions; red currants; fresh flat-leaf parsley

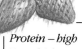

Protein – high
Fat – high
Fiber – high

Summer Vegetables with Wild Rice

⅓ cup	white rice
⅓ cup	brown rice
¼ cup	wild rice
1 head cauliflower, broken into florets	
½ lb	zucchini, diced
½ cup	green beans, cut in 1-inch lengths
½ cup	peas, fresh or frozen
1 tbsp	lemon juice
2 tbsp	polyunsaturated margarine
salt and freshly ground pepper	

Sauce

2 tbsp	polyunsaturated margarine
2 tbsp	flour
1 cup	low-fat milk
2 oz	Parmesan cheese, grated
2 tsp	chopped fresh parsley
2 tsp	pesto sauce
1 tsp	sesame seeds, toasted

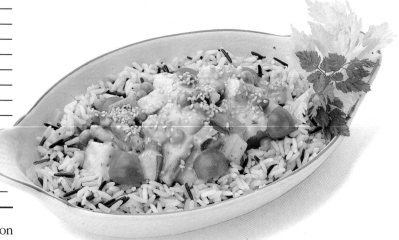

Prepare and cook each type of rice according to the instructions on the packet. Meanwhile, steam the vegetables until just tender. Remove from the heat and toss with the lemon juice, margarine and seasoning.

To make the sauce, melt the margarine, stir in the flour and cook gently for 1–2 minutes. Gradually add the milk and heat, stirring constantly, until the sauce thickens. Allow to cook, then add half the Parmesan cheese, and all the parsley and pesto sauce.

To serve, drain the white, brown and wild rice and mix them together. Arrange in a serving dish. Pile the vegetables on top. Cover with the sauce and sprinkle with the remaining Parmesan mixed with sesame seeds. Lightly brown under the broiler.

Variations

Replace the rice with a wholewheat pasta.

Substitute other vegetables in season.

Garnish cherry tomatoes; celery top; fresh chervil

Protein – medium
Fat – medium
Fiber – medium

Flan(s)
    Gardener's Delight 41
    Nutty Vegetable Flan 90
Flours, choice of 5
Fresh Herb Oatcakes 91
Ful medame beans 4

Garbanzo Fritters 37
Garden Pizza 61
Gardener's Delight 41
Garlic Butter 56
Garlic Sauce 8
Garnish, importance of 1
Garnishes 99
Grains 2
Green peas 4
Gumbo Stew 14

Haricot beans 4
    Gumbo Stew 14
    Haricot and Potato Pie 44
Haricot and Potato Pie 44
Harvest Burger 66
Harvest Crumble 13
Harvest Pancakes 16
Herb Oatcakes, Fresh 91
Herbs, fresh 1, 5
Hot Crudité! 8
"Hot" Peppers 30

Indonesian-style Vegetables 92
Italian-style Peppers 19

Kebab with Nut Risotto 60
Kidney beans 4

Chilli sin Carne 62

Lemon and Millet Hotpot 75
Lentil and Cauliflower Spice 23
Lentil Duchesse 24
Lentil Moussaka 53
Lentil Pilaf 76
Lentil Roast 11
Lentil Turnovers 87
Lentils 4
    Delhi Lasagne 10
    Dhal 70
    Lentil and Cauliflower Spice 23
    Lentil Duchesse 24
    Lentil Moussaka 53
    Lentil Pilaf 76
    Lentil Roast 11
    Lentil Turnovers 87
    Wholemeal Lentil Pancakes 81
Lima Bean Curry 34
Lima beans – see butter beans

Macaroni Crisp 55
Mexican Chickpeas 57
Midwinter Pie 89
Millet 102
    Lemon and Millet Hotpot 75
Mung beans 4
Mushroom Crunch 31
Mushroom Envelopes 63
Mushroom Omelette 39

Nuts 2
Nutty Burgers 38
Nutty Hotpot with Cheese Dumplings 71

Nutty Vegetable Flans 90

Okra 102
Omelette Collection 39
Onion clouté 102

Pancakes
    Fillings for 16
    Harvest 16
    Soufflé 12
    Wholemeal Lentil 81
Parsley Sauce 81
Parsnips
    Croquettes Mont Blanc 33
Pasta
    Canneloni Verdi 15
    Cheese and Vegetable Macaroni 86
    Chickpeas Provençale 20
    Chinese Vegetables with Pasta 83
    Delhi Lasagne 10
    Macaroni Crisp 55
    Pasta del Bria 47
    Singapore Stroganoff 18
    Spinach and Blue Cheese Lasagne 67
    Vegetable Fusilli 78
Pasta del Bria 47
Pasta Omelette 39
Peppers
    Capsicum and Chickpea Couscous 35
    "Hot" Peppers 30
    Italian-style Peppers 19
    Ratatouille 32
    stuffed, preparation of 5
Pinto beans 4
Potato Medley 69

Potatoes
    Haricot and Potato Pie 44
    Indonesian-style Vegetables 92
    Midwinter Pie 89
    Potato Medley 69
    Swiss Potato Croquettes 65
Protein 2

"Quick" Tomato Sauce 97

Ratatouille 32
Red kidney beans – see kidney beans
Refresh, to 103
Rice
    Cashew Paella 9
    Risotto 60
    Summer Vegetables with Wild Rice 42
    Suppli 22
    Sweet 'n' Sour Rissoles 45
Ricotta 103
Risotto 60
Roux 103

Sag Madras 64
Sandwiches, Vegetarian 100–101
Sauces 96–98
Scallion Fleuron 99, 103
Seeds 2
Sesame seeds 103
Singapore Stroganoff 18
Soufflé Filling 12
Soufflé Pancakes 12
Soy beans 4
Spanish Omelette 39
Spinach and Blue Cheese Lasagne 67

Spinach and Cheese Omelette 39
Spinach Roulade 79
Summer Vegetables with Wild Rice 42
Suppli 22
Sweet 'n' Savory Loaf 54
Sweet 'n' Sour Rissoles 45
Sweet 'n' Sour Vegetables 52
Swiss Potato Croquettes 65

Tofu 103
Tomato Sauce 96
Tomatoes
    "Quick" Tomato Sauce 97
    Ratatouille 32
    Tomato Sauce 96

Vegetable Cheesecake 21
Vegetable Fusilli 78
Vegetable Stir-fry 58
Vegetable stock 5
Vegetable Symphony 88
Vegetable Tortilla 74
Vegetarian diet 1, 2
Vegetarian Sandwiches 100–101

Walnut and Roquefort Savory 84
White Béchamel 96
    cheese 96
    lentil 96
    mint 96
    mushroom 96
    onion 96
    spinach 96
    yogurt 96
Wholemeal Lentil Pancakes 81

Wholesome Hotpot 26
Wild Green Risotto 25
Wild rice 103
Winter Cobbler 80

Yogurt sauce, hot, to prevent separation 5

Zucchini
    Canneloni Verdi 15
    Eggplant and Zucchini Bake 27
    Ratatouille 32
    Summer Vegetables with Wild Rice 42
    Vegetable Symphony 88
    Zucchini Crunch 48

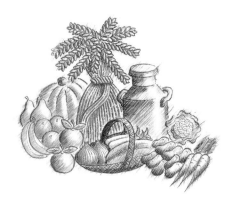

"Crisp" Savory Cheesecake

Crust	
1 oz	plain unsalted potato chips
4 oz	wholewheat bran crackers
1/4 cup	chopped mixed nuts
6 tbsp	polyunsaturated margarine

Topping	
4 oz	blue cheese, softened
4 oz	low-fat cream cheese, softened
1 tsp	mustard
1 tsp	snipped fresh chives
	salt and freshly ground pepper
3/4 cup	heavy cream, lightly whipped

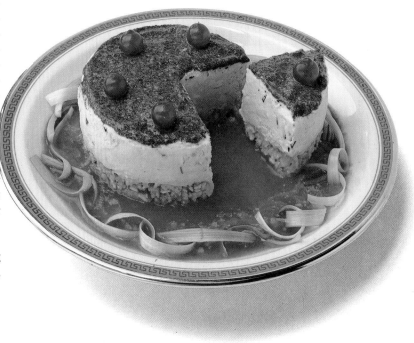

To prepare the crust, crush the potato chips and crackers until they resemble fine crumbs. Mix in the nuts. Melt the margarine, add the crumbs and mix well. Press the mixture into one large or four individual flan dishes. Chill.

Beat the cheeses together. Add the mustard, chives and seasoning and mix. Stir in the cream, blending well. Turn out onto the crust, level with a knife and chill until set.

Serve topped with spinach purée on a tomato coulis (see page 102).

Garnish scallion shavings; cranberries; finely ground nuts

Protein – medium
Fat – high
Fiber – medium

Haricot and Potato Pie

½ cup	dried haricot beans
½ cup	chopped onions
1 clove garlic, finely chopped	
1 tbsp	polyunsaturated oil
1 lb	zucchini, sliced
¾ cup	vegetable stock
⅔ cup	canned tomatoes, chopped
2 tbsp	tomato purée
2 tbsp	low-fat milk
2 tbsp	scallion, finely chopped
1 lb	whipped potatoes
salt and freshly ground pepper	

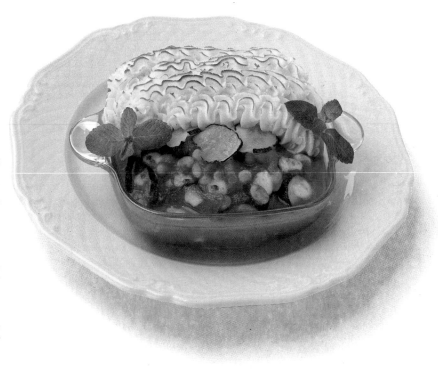

Soak the haricot beans overnight (see page 4). Drain, rinse and place in a pot of cold water. Bring to a boil and cook rapidly for 10 minutes. Reduce the heat and simmer for about 1 hour. Drain. Alternatively use 1½ cups canned or cooked haricot beans.

Sauté the onion and garlic in the oil. Add the zucchini, stock, tomatoes, tomato purée and seasoning and bring to a boil. Simmer for 10 minutes. Add the beans and place in an ovenproof dish.

Beat the milk, scallion, salt and pepper into the whipped potatoes. Spread or pipe the mixture over the vegetables and bake at 350°F for 30–40 minutes.

Variation
Use different types of beans and vary the base vegetable.

Garnish sliced zucchini; fresh mint leaves

Protein – low
Fat – low
Fiber – high

Sweet 'n' Sour Rissoles

1 cup	brown rice
2 tbsp	polyunsaturated margarine
1/2 cup	chopped onions
2 tbsp	wholemeal breadcrumbs
1 cup	walnuts, finely ground
1/2 tsp	chopped fresh thyme
1/2 tsp	chopped fresh sage
1/2 cup	canned tomatoes, chopped
1 tsp	soy sauce
	1 egg, beaten
	polyunsaturated oil
Sauce	
1/2 cup	canned apples
	pinch ground cinnamon

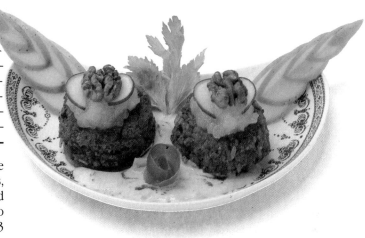

Cook the rice and refresh well with cold water. Melt the margarine and sauté the onion until soft. Mix with the rice, breadcrumbs, walnuts and herbs. Combine with the tomatoes and soy sauce and sufficient egg to bind, adding more breadcrumbs if the texture is too moist. Shape the mixture into rissoles. Shallow-fry in oil for 3 minutes on each side.

To make the sauce, purée the apples, add the cinnamon and heat gently.

Serve the rissoles hot with green vegetables or a salad, accompanied by the apple sauce.

Garnish sauce of plain yogurt and pesto; puréed apple flavored with honey; feathered apples (see page 99); tomato rose; celery tops; radish slices; walnut halves

Protein – low
Fat – high
Fiber – medium

Eggplant Parcels

½ cup   lentils
½ lb   eggplant, diced
1   onion, chopped
4 tbsp   polyunsaturated oil
1   red pepper, seeded and diced
1 tsp   ground cumin
1 tsp   ground cinnamon
1 tsp   curry paste
salt and freshly ground pepper
4 oz   Caerphilly cheese, diced
2 tsp   chopped fresh oregano
½ lb   filo pastry
1 egg
2 tbsp   low-fat milk

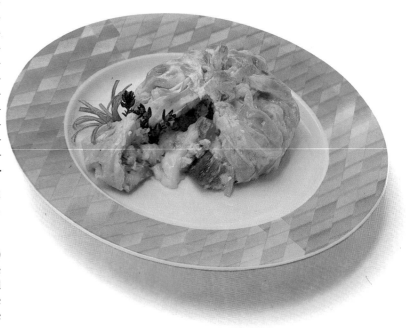

Soak the lentils as required (see page 4). Drain, rinse and place in a pot of cold water. Bring to a boil and cook rapidly for 10 minutes. Reduce the heat and simmer for 20–30 minutes. Drain and cool.

Sprinkle the eggplant with salt and allow to drain in a colander for 30 minutes. Rinse thoroughly and dry, using paper toweling. Sauté the onion in half the oil until soft. Add the eggplant and red pepper and cook for 2–3 minutes. Stir in the spices and curry paste and continue to cook for an additional 2 minutes. Season and let cool. Stir in the lentils, cheese and oregano.

To make the parcels: place one layer of filo pastry on a work surface. Brush with water. Lay a second layer on top and brush with water. Cut into four 6-inch squares. Brush all the edges of the pastry with water. Mound a portion of the eggplant mixture in the center of each square. Fold up the corners and sides of the pastry to form a parcel shape. Beat the egg with the milk and egg wash the parcels. Place on a greased baking pan and cook at 325°F for 30 minutes, or until the pastry is golden-brown. Serve hot or cold.

Variation
Substitute artichoke hearts for the eggplant.

Garnish scallion fleuron (see page 99); fresh thyme

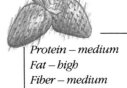

Protein – medium
Fat – high
Fiber – medium

Pasta del Bria

6 oz	pasta shapes (egg, spinach and tomato)
1 lb	cauliflower, broken into florets
1¼ cups	sliced leeks
1¼ cups	sliced flat or button mushrooms
4 tbsp	polyunsaturated margarine
¼ cup	flour
2 cups	low-fat milk
	salt and freshly ground pepper
6 oz	low-fat Cheddar cheese, grated

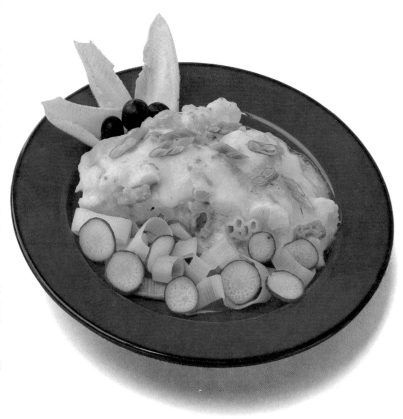

Cook the pasta in boiling, salted water until just tender. Drain, refresh in cold water, and set aside.

Cook the cauliflower and leeks in boiling, salted water until just tender. Drain well, put in an ovenproof dish and keep warm. Cook the mushrooms in their own juices, drain and add to the cauliflower and leeks.

To prepare the sauce, melt the margarine, stir in the flour and cook for 1–2 minutes. Gradually add the milk and seasoning and bring to a boil, stirring constantly. Allow the sauce to cook. Stir in the pasta and half of the cheese. Slowly bring the mixture back to a boil.

Pour the sauce over the vegetables, sprinkle with the remaining cheese and place under the broiler until golden-brown.

Variation
Mix sesame seeds with grated cheese to provide a more unusual topping.

Garnish leek shavings; sliced radish; chicory leaves; sliced scallions; black olives

Protein – high
Fat – medium
Fiber – high

Zucchini Crunch

1 tbsp polyunsaturated oil
1/2 cup chopped onions
1 clove garlic, finely chopped
1 lb zucchini, canelled (see page 102) and thinly sliced
salt and freshly ground pepper
2 cups canned tomatoes, chopped
2 tbsp tomato purée
2 tbsp polyunsaturated margarine
2 tbsp flour
1 cup low-fat milk
1/4 cup wholemeal breadcrumbs, toasted
3 oz low-fat Cheddar cheese, grated
2 tsp chopped fresh mixed herbs (oregano, thyme, chives and basil)
1/4 cup chopped mixed nuts

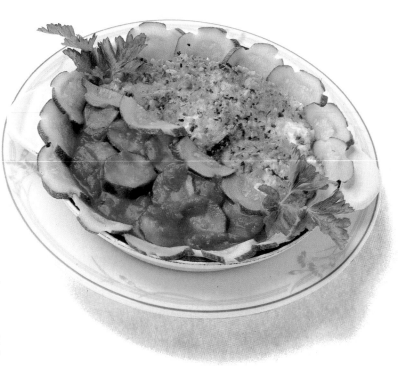

Heat the oil and sauté the onions and garlic until soft. Add the zucchini and seasoning and cook for 5 minutes. Add the tomatoes and tomato purée, and a little water or vegetable stock if required. Simmer for about 10 minutes, until the zucchini is just cooked.

To prepare the white sauce, melt the margarine, add the flour and cook gently for 1–2 minutes. Gradually add the milk and heat, stirring constantly, until the sauce thickens. Allow to cook.

Transfer the vegetables to a serving dish. Cover with the sauce. Mix the breadcrumbs, cheese, herbs and nuts together and sprinkle over the top. Place under the broiler until brown and bubbling.

Garnish sliced zucchini; fresh flat-leaf parsley

Protein – medium
Fat – high
Fiber – low

Eggplant Layer

1½ lb	eggplant, cut into ½-inch slices
¼ lb	zucchini, sliced
4 tbsp	polyunsaturated oil
½ cup	finely diced onions
½ cup	diced sweet peppers
1 clove garlic, finely chopped	
1 tsp	fennel seeds
½ tsp	chopped fresh oregano
2 cups	canned tomatoes, chopped
salt and freshly ground pepper	
½ lb	Mozzarella cheese, thinly sliced
½ cup	wholemeal breadcrumbs
2 oz	Parmesan cheese, grated

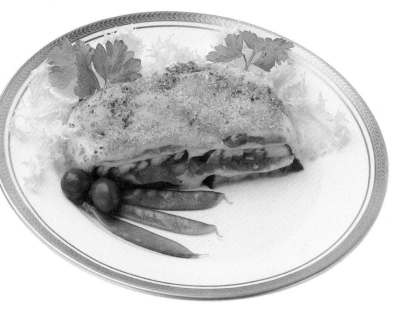

Sprinkle the eggplant slices with salt and allow to drain. Dry slices and brush both sides with a little oil. Place on a baking pan and bake at 400°F for 30–45 minutes, until lightly browned and tender. Blanch and refresh the zucchini.

Meanwhile, make a thick tomato sauce. Heat the oil and sauté the onions, but do not allow to turn brown. Add the peppers, garlic, fennel seeds, oregano, tomatoes, a little water and seasoning. Bring to a boil and simmer for 30 minutes.

In an ovenproof dish, place a layer of eggplant and zucchini, and top with a layer of tomato sauce and Mozzarella. Repeat layers, finishing with the Mozzarella. Combine the breadcrumbs and Parmesan cheese and sprinkle generously over the top. Bake at 375°F for 30 minutes.

Garnish endive; fresh flat-leaf parsley; cranberries

Protein – medium
Fat – high
Fiber – high

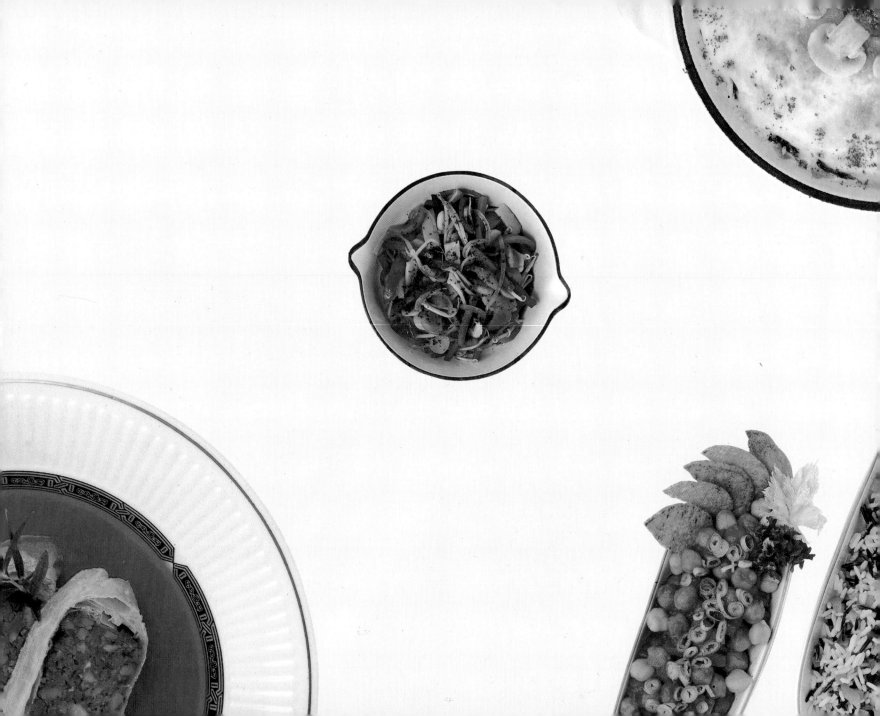

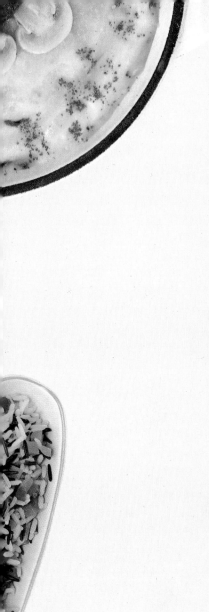

The
AUTUMN
collection

Twenty delicious dishes without meat

Sweet 'n' Sour Vegetables

6 oz	potatoes, cut into 1 × ½-inch sticks
½ cup	carrots, canelled (see page 102) and sliced
¼ lb	zucchini, canelled (see page 102) and sliced
⅓ cup	diced dessert apple
½ cup	red pepper, cut into 1 × ½-inch sticks
1 cup	vegetable stock
1 cup	sliced mushrooms
⅓ cup	canned tomatoes, chopped
⅓ cup	water chestnuts, sliced

Sauce

1 tbsp	polyunsaturated oil
½ cup	chopped onions
1 clove garlic, finely chopped
1 tbsp	tomato purée
1 tbsp	soy sauce
2 tbsp	white wine vinegar
1 tbsp	dry sherry (optional)
1 tsp	ground ginger
2 tbsp	brown sugar
1 tbsp	chopped mixed nuts
salt and freshly ground pepper
1 tbsp	arrowroot

Reserve some vegetables to blanch for garnish. Cook the potatoes, carrots, zucchini, apple and red pepper in a little of the stock for 10 minutes, until just tender. In a separate pan, soften the mushrooms and tomatoes in a little more stock. Add to the other vegetables with the water chestnuts.

In a large pan or wok, heat the oil and gently cook the onion and garlic.

Combine the remaining sauce ingredients except the arrowroot with the remaining stock and add to the onion and garlic, stirring well. Blend the arrowroot with a little water and add to the sauce.

Add the vegetables to the sauce, stir and bring to a boil. Reduce the heat and simmer for 5 minutes. Serve with a mixture of long-grain white rice and wild rice.

Variation
Serve with noodles or as a filling for baked potatoes.

Garnish blanched vegetables; chopped fresh parsley

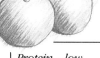

Protein – low
Fat – low
Fiber – low

Lentil Moussaka

½ cup	lentils
4 tbsp	polyunsaturated oil
½ cup	chopped onions
1 clove garlic, finely chopped	
1¼ cups	sliced mushrooms
½ cup	vegetable stock
2 tbsp	tomato purée
1 tsp	chopped fresh oregano
salt and freshly ground pepper	
½ tsp	ground nutmeg
¾ lb	eggplant, sliced, salted and drained
2 tomatoes, skinned and sliced	
2 potatoes, boiled and sliced	

Sauce

2 tbsp	polyunsaturated margarine
2 tbsp	flour
1 cup	low-fat milk
2 oz	low-fat Cheddar cheese, grated
pinch dry mustard	
salt and freshly ground pepper	

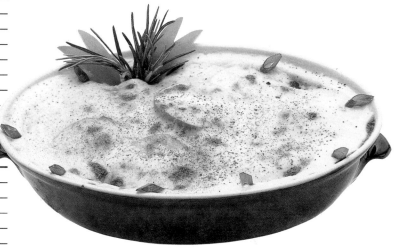

Soak the lentils as required (see page 4). Drain, rinse and place in a pot of cold water. Bring to a boil and cook rapidly for 10 minutes. Reduce the heat and simmer for 20–30 minutes.

Heat 2 tbsp of the oil and sauté the onions and garlic gently. Add the mushrooms and lentils and cook for a few more minutes. Mix in the stock, tomato purée and oregano. Season well, add the nutmeg and remove from the heat. Sauté the eggplant slices in the remaining oil until soft.

Spread the lentil mixture over the bottom of an oiled ovenproof dish, cover with the eggplant slices, then a layer of tomato slices and top with the potato slices.

To make the sauce, melt the margarine, add the flour and cook gently for 1–2 minutes. Gradually add the milk and stir over a low heat until the sauce thickens. Allow to cook before adding half of the cheese and the mustard. Season. Pour the sauce over the moussaka and sprinkle with the remaining cheese.
Bake at 350°F for 20 minutes, or until the cheese is golden-brown and bubbling.

Variation
Replace the lentils with cooked mixed beans.

Garnish fresh rosemary; tomato; chopped scallion tops

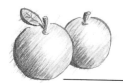

Protein – medium
Fat – high
Fiber – high

Sweet 'n' Savory Loaf

1 cup	finely chopped peanuts
¾ cup	grated carrots
¾ cup	finely chopped celery
⅓ cup	grated dessert apple
⅓ cup	wholemeal breadcrumbs
1 tsp	chopped fresh mixed herbs (thyme, basil, oregano and sage)
	salt and freshly ground pepper
1 egg	
¼ cup	low-fat milk
2 tsp	tomato purée

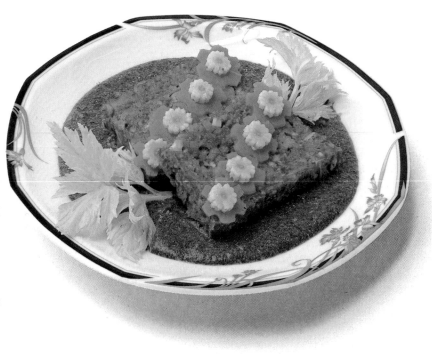

Mix the peanuts, carrots, celery, apple, breadcrumbs, herbs and seasoning. Combine with the egg, milk and tomato purée, and mix thoroughly. If the mixture is too moist, add more breadcrumbs. Press the mixture into a greased 1-lb loaf pan or individual pudding molds and bake at 350°F for 30–35 minutes.

Turn out and serve with a spinach sauce (see page 96).

Variations
To make a more substantial dish, combine the ingredients with cooked brown rice. Cook as above but serve from the pan.

Serve with a tomato sauce.

Garnish carrot slices; baby sweetcorn slices; celery tops

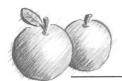

Protein – low
Fat – medium
Fiber – medium

Macaroni Crisp

2 tbsp	polyunsaturated margarine
½ cup	chopped onions
1 clove garlic, finely chopped	
2 cups	canned tomatoes, chopped
1 tsp	chopped fresh oregano
salt and freshly ground pepper	
2½ cups	broccoli florets
4 oz	wholewheat or egg macaroni
1 cup	plain yogurt
2 oz	Roquefort cheese
1 oz	Mozzarella cheese
2 tbsp	rolled oats

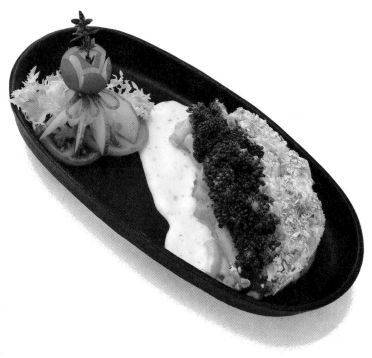

Melt the margarine and sauté the onions and garlic. Add the tomatoes, oregano, 1 cup of cold water and seasoning and simmer for about 20 minutes. Cook the broccoli in boiling, salted water until just tender; drain and refresh in cold water. In a separate pan, cook the macaroni in boiling water for 10–15 minutes, until just tender; drain and refresh in cold water.

In an ovenproof dish, layer half the tomato sauce and macaroni. Add the broccoli. Repeat the layers of sauce and macaroni.

Beat the yogurt and cheeses together, spread over the macaroni and sprinkle evenly with the oats. Bake at 400°F for 30 minutes, or until the top is lightly browned.

Serve with a light mint-flavored Béchamel (see page 96).

Variations
Replace the broccoli with another vegetable, such as cauliflower or zucchini.

Use wholewheat pasta shapes instead of the macaroni.

Garnish sliced tomato; endive; fan of cucumber slices; radish flower; fresh thyme

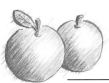

Protein – *medium*
Fat – *medium*
Fiber – *medium*

Butter Bean Kiev

1 cup   dried butter beans
⅔ cup   wholemeal breadcrumbs
salt and freshly ground pepper
2 tbsp   polyunsaturated margarine
1 onion, diced
1 egg
2 tbsp   low-fat milk
polyunsaturated oil
Garlic Butter
6 tbsp   butter
2 cloves garlic, finely chopped
1 tsp   chopped fresh parsley

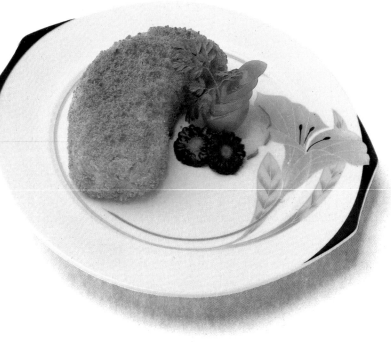

Soak the butter beans overnight (see page 3). Drain, rinse, and place in a pot of cold water. Bring to a boil and cook rapidly for 10 minutes. Reduce the heat and simmer for about 1½ hours. Drain. Alternatively use 3 cups canned or cooked butter beans.

To prepare the garlic butter, soften the butter and blend in the garlic and parsley. Roll in wax paper and chill until firm.

Mash the butter beans and mix in half of the breadcrumbs and seasoning. Melt the margarine and sauté the onion until soft, but do not allow to turn brown. Add the onion to the butter bean mixture and mix well. Shape the mixture into four cutlets. Place a cube or slice of garlic butter in the center of each cutlet, and mold the mixture around it.

Lightly beat the egg with the milk. Egg wash each cutlet and coat with the remaining breadcrumbs. Sauté each side of the cutlets until golden-brown. Alternatively, broil or bake the cutlets, turning once. Serve with a selection of chutneys.

Variations
Use any other cooked bean as the base of the cutlets.

Replace the garlic butter with an herb- or lemon-flavored butter, or slices of cheese.

Garnish feathered tomato; cucumber; fresh chervil; sliced black currant

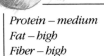

Protein – medium
Fat – high
Fiber – high

Mexican Chickpeas

³/₄ cup   dried chickpeas
1 tbsp   polyunsaturated oil
¹/₂ cup   finely chopped onions
¹/₂ tsp   chilli powder
1 tsp   ground cumin
2 red or green peppers, finely chopped
2 tbsp   tomato purée
1¹/₂ cups   vegetable stock
lemon juice
salt and freshly ground pepper

Soak the chickpeas overnight (see page 4). Drain, rinse, and place in a pot of cold water. Bring to a boil and cook rapidly for 10 minutes. Reduce the heat and simmer for 1–1¹/₂ hours. Alternatively use 2 cups canned or cooked chickpeas.

Heat the oil in a large pan and sauté the onions and spices gently for 5 minutes. Add the peppers and chickpeas and stir. Combine the tomato purée with the stock and add to the vegetables. Stir well and cook for 10 minutes. Add seasoning and a little lemon juice.

Serve with a mixture of white, brown and wild rice combined with finely diced red and green peppers.

Variation
Serve with wholewheat pasta or toasted pita bread and a crisp salad.

Garnish tortilla chips; scallions; celery top; red leaf lettuce

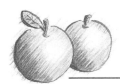

Protein – low
Fat – medium
Fiber – high

Vegetable Stir-fry

1 tbsp   polyunsaturated oil
½ cup   sliced onions
1 clove garlic, finely chopped
2 medium carrots, cut into sticks
½ green pepper, cut into sticks
¼ lb   broccoli, broken into small florets
¼ lb   baby sweetcorn
¾ cup   chopped tomatoes
3 tbsp   cider vinegar
2 tbsp   brown sugar
1 cup   pineapple juice
1 vegetable stock cube, crumbled
2 tsp   soy sauce
1 tsp   ground ginger
salt and freshly ground pepper
½ cup   bamboo shoots
⅓ cup   sliced water chestnuts
1 tbsp   arrowroot

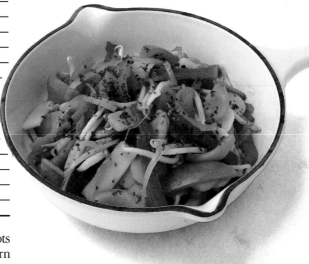

Heat the oil in a large pan or wok. Add the onion, garlic and carrots and sauté until the onion is soft. Add the pepper, broccoli, sweetcorn and tomatoes. Combine the vinegar, sugar, pineapple juice, crumbled stock cube and soy sauce and pour over the vegetables. Add the ginger, a little water and seasoning and stir well. Bring to a boil, reduce the heat, cover and simmer, skimming occasionally until the vegetables are tender but still crisp.

Stir in the bamboo shoots and water chestnuts. Blend the arrowroot with a little water, add to the stir-fry, mix well and cook for an additional 2 minutes. Serve immediately.

Variations
Serve the stir-fry with brown rice or wholewheat noodles.

Use the stir-fry as a filling for pancakes, or as a layer in a nut roast.

Garnish chopped fresh parsley

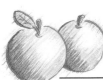

Protein – low
Fat – low
Fiber – low

Chickpeas Wellington

²/₃ cup	dried chickpeas
2 tsp	yeast extract
5 oz	Brazil nuts, ground
²/₃ cup	wholemeal breadcrumbs
¹/₂ cup	finely chopped onions
2 cups	sliced mushrooms
	vegetable stock
2 tsp	chopped fresh mixed herbs
	salt and freshly ground pepper
¹/₂ lb	flaky pastry
1 egg	
2 tbsp	low-fat milk

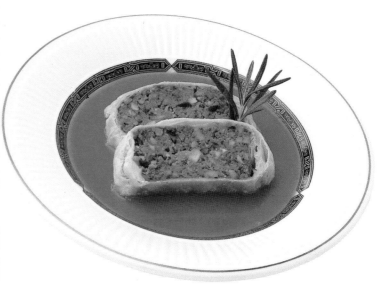

Soak the chickpeas overnight (see page 4). Drain, rinse and place in a pot of cold water. Bring to a boil and cook rapidly for 10 minutes. Reduce the heat and simmer for about 1½ hours. Alternatively use 2 cups canned or cooked chickpeas.

Place the chickpeas, yeast extract, Brazil nuts and breadcrumbs in a food processor and blend. Sauté the onions and mushrooms until they produce their own liquid, then add the chickpea mixture to the pan, adding sufficient vegetable stock to obtain a firm mixture. Add the herbs and seasonings and mix thoroughly.

Mold the mixture into a loaf shape. Roll out the flaky pastry and use to wrap the loaf, covering it completely. Beat the egg and milk together and egg wash the pastry. Bake at 400°F for 20–30 minutes, or until the pastry is crisp and lightly browned.

Serve with tomato sauce (see page 96).

Variations
Replace the Brazil nuts with other types of nuts.

Serve with an apple or cranberry sauce.

Garnish tomato coulis (page 102); fresh rosemary

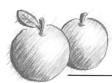

Protein – high
Fat – high
Fiber – high

Kebab with Nut Risotto

For each Kebab	
2 chunks red onion	
2 chunks red pepper	
5 slices zucchini	
3 button mushrooms	
2 chunks green pepper	
2 cherry tomatoes	
2 tbsp polyunsaturated margarine, melted	
Risotto (serves 4)	
4 tbsp polyunsaturated margarine	
1 cup long-grain brown rice	
2 cups boiling water	
1¼ cups thinly sliced mushrooms	
⅓ cup cooked peas	
½ cup halved roasted peanuts	
or	
½ cup roughly chopped walnuts	
2 oz Parmesan cheese, grated	
1 tbsp lemon juice	
salt and freshly ground pepper	

Thread a chunk of onion, a chunk of red pepper, a slice of zucchini, a mushroom, a chunk of green pepper and a tomato on a kebab stick or long skewer; repeat. Brush the vegetables with margarine and broil, turning frequently, for about 10 minutes.

To make the risotto, melt the margarine and sauté the rice gently for a few minutes. Add the boiling water and cook the rice for 25–30 minutes, or until tender; most of the water should have been absorbed. Stir in the sliced mushrooms, peas, nuts and grated cheese and heat through for 5 minutes. Add the lemon juice and seasoning.

Serve the kebabs and risotto with barbecue sauce (see page 98).

Variation
Consider other combinations for the kebabs, such as tofu, artichoke hearts and eggplant.

Garnish red chicory; Chinese cabbage; fresh rosemary; fresh flat-leaf parsley

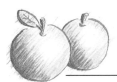

Protein – medium
Fat – high
Fiber – medium

Garden Pizza

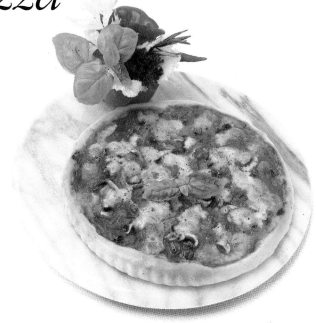

Crust
2 packages dry active yeast
3 tbsp warm water
¾ cup wholemeal flour
pinch baking powder
2 tbsp polyunsaturated margarine
3 tbsp low-fat milk

Topping
½ cup finely diced onions
1 clove garlic, finely chopped
1 tbsp polyunsaturated oil
⅓ cup tomato purée
1 cup canned tomatoes, chopped
pinch fresh chopped basil
pinch fresh chopped oregano
½ cup diced sweet peppers
1 cup sliced mushrooms
⅓ cup canned artichokes, sliced (optional)
5 oz Mozzarella cheese, diced

Dissolve the yeast in the warm water and set aside until it foams. Meanwhile, sift the flour and baking powder. Cut the margarine into small cubes, add to the flour and gently fold in. Stir in the milk and yeast mixture and mix to a stiff dough. Knead lightly and allow to rise for 30 minutes. Roll out the dough to a ½-inch thickness and slightly loosen the edges.

To make the topping: sauté the onions and garlic in the oil. Add the tomato purée, chopped tomatoes and herbs and simmer for 15 minutes. Season generously. Meanwhile, lightly sauté the peppers and mushrooms.

Spread the tomato sauce on the crust. Arrange the peppers and mushrooms and top with sliced artichokes. Sprinkle with the cheese. Bake the pizza at 450°F for 15–18 minutes.

Variations
Experiment with different toppings and try making individual pizzas.

Use a different flour or add ingredients such as oats, herbs, garlic or chopped spinach to the dough, or, for speed, use a pizza dough mix.

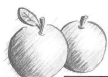

Garnish red pepper; red leaf lettuce; Chinese cabbage; celery top; fresh basil; fresh rosemary; red chilli

Protein – high
Fat – medium
Fiber – medium

Chilli Sin Carne

²/₃ cup	dried kidney beans
1 tbsp	polyunsaturated oil
1 cup	chopped onions
1 red pepper, diced	
1 green pepper, diced	
1 stalk celery, diced	
15 oz	canned tomatoes, chopped
2 tbsp	tomato purée
½ tsp	chilli powder
pinch cayenne	
½ tsp	ground cumin
1 tsp	chopped fresh oregano
salt and freshly ground pepper	
1 cup	vegetable stock

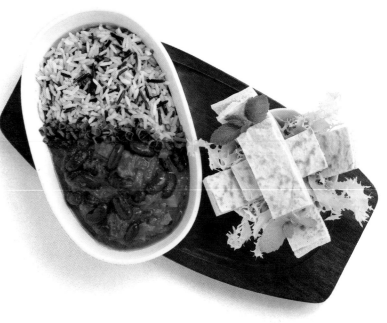

Soak the kidney beans overnight (see page 4). Drain, rinse and place in a pot of cold water. Bring to a boil and cook rapidly for 10 minutes. Reduce the heat and simmer for about 1 hour. Drain. Alternatively use 2 cups canned or cooked kidney beans.

Heat the oil and sauté the onion, peppers and celery until tender. Add the beans, tomatoes, tomato purée, chilli powder, cayenne, cumin and oregano. Season well. Add the stock and simmer for about 30 minutes, until the flavors blend and the chilli thickens slightly.

Serve with a mixture of white, brown and wild rice.

Variations
Stuff green peppers with chilli sin carne and bake until peppers are tender.

Use as a baked potato topping.

Serve topped with sour cream or guacamole.

Use as a turnover filling.

Garnish snipped fresh chives; sliced pita bread; endive; fresh mint

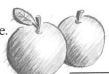

Protein – medium
Fat – low
Fiber – high

Mushroom Envelopes

1 tbsp	polyunsaturated oil
1 cup	finely chopped onions
1 clove garlic, finely chopped	
2¹/₂ cups	sliced mushrooms
1 tsp	chopped fresh mixed herbs (basil, chives, oregano and thyme)
pinch cayenne	
3 eggs, hard-boiled	
salt and freshly ground pepper	
¹/₂ lb	puff pastry
1 egg	
2 tbsp	low-fat milk

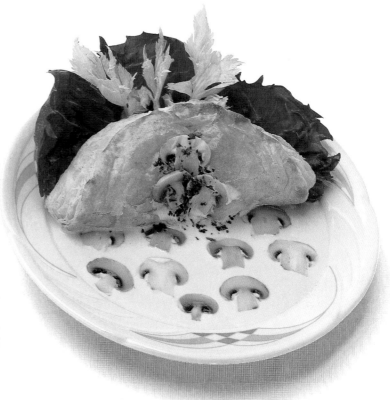

Heat the oil and sauté the onion and garlic for 3–4 minutes, then add the mushrooms, herbs and cayenne. Cover and cook just until tender. Remove from the heat and cool.

Separate the hard-boiled eggs. Mash the yolks, chop the whites and add both to the mushroom mixture. Season.

Roll out the pastry and cut into four 6-inch circles. Beat the egg and milk together and use to brush the edges of the pastry. Spoon 1–2 tablespoons of the filling into the center of each pastry circle, fold the pastry over and seal the edges. Brush each pastry with the egg wash, pierce a hole in the top and bake at 425°F for 15–20 minutes.

Serve with mushroom sauce (see page 96).

Variation
Use a wholemeal pastry, which will give a heavier texture to the envelopes.

Garnish radicchio; celery tops; sliced mushrooms; chopped fresh parsley

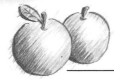

Protein – low
Fat – high
Fiber – low

Sag Madras

⅓ cup   dried chickpeas
2 tbsp   polyunsaturated margarine
½ cup   chopped onions
1 clove garlic, finely chopped
1 tsp   turmeric
1 tsp   ground coriander
½ tsp   ground ginger
1 tsp   garam masala (Indian seasoning)
1 tbsp   mild curry powder
½ lb   potatoes, cubed
1 cup   vegetable stock
1 tbsp   tomato purée
½ lb   fresh leaf spinach
¾ cup   canned tomatoes, chopped
2 cups   sliced mushrooms
salt and freshly ground pepper

Soak chickpeas overnight (see page 4). Drain, rinse and place in a pot of cold water. Bring to a boil and cook rapidly for 10 minutes. Reduce the heat and simmer for about 1½ hours. Drain. Alternatively use 1 cup canned or cooked chickpeas.

Melt the margarine and sauté the onions and garlic. Add the spices and cook for 2 minutes. Add the potatoes, chickpeas, stock and tomato purée and simmer for 15 minutes. Add the remaining ingredients and simmer for an additional 10 minutes.

Serve with brown rice and naan bread. Yogurt would make a refreshing accompaniment.

Garnish radish rose; fresh parsley;
scallion fleuron (see page 99); chopped
scallions

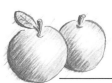

Protein – low
Fat – medium
Fiber – medium

Swiss Potato Croquettes

1 lb	potatoes
4 tbsp	polyunsaturated margarine
2 eggs	
pinch ground nutmeg	
salt and freshly ground pepper	
⅓ cup	wholemeal breadcrumbs
2 tsp	chopped fresh mixed herbs (oregano, basil, chives and thyme)
1 oz	Parmesan cheese, grated
¼ lb	Gruyère cheese, diced
2 tbsp	flour

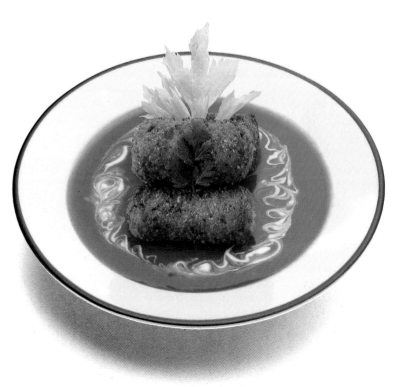

Boil and mash the potatoes. Add the margarine, 1 egg, the nutmeg and seasonings and mix well. Allow to cool. Meanwhile, mix the breadcrumbs, herbs and Parmesan cheese. Beat the remaining egg.

Shape the potato mixture into croquettes, putting some diced Gruyère in the center of each one. Dip the croquettes first in the flour, then the beaten egg and finally the breadcrumb mixture. Bake on an oiled baking pan at 350°F for about 30 minutes, until golden-brown, turning once. Alternatively, deep-fry the croquettes for 2–3 minutes.

Serve with a spicy sauce, such as hot barbecue (see page 98), laced with plain yogurt, or chilled yogurt flavored with mint.

Garnish celery tops; fresh chervil

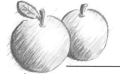

Protein – medium
Fat – high
Fiber – medium

Harvest Burger

⅔ cup   dried mixed beans (eg: kidney, black-eyed and haricot)
1 tbsp   polyunsaturated oil
½ cup   finely chopped onions
1 clove garlic, finely chopped
½ cup   vegetable stock
2 tbsp   tomato purée
1 tsp   chopped fresh mixed herbs (oregano, thyme, chives and basil)
1 tsp   paprika
salt and freshly ground pepper
2 tbsp   wholemeal flour
2 oz   Mozzarella cheese, sliced
2 tomatoes, sliced
4 burger buns

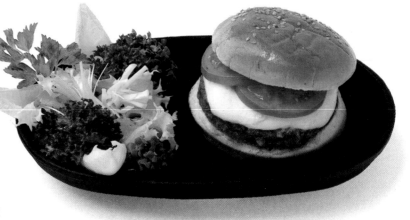

Soak the beans overnight (see page 3). Drain, rinse and place in 3 separate pots of cold water. Bring to a boil and cook rapidly for 10 minutes. Reduce the heat and simmer for the required time. Drain. Alternatively use 2 cups canned or cooked beans.

Heat the oil and sauté the onion and garlic until soft. Add the stock and bring to a boil. Add the beans, tomato purée, herbs, paprika and seasonings. Simmer the mixture until the liquid has evaporated.

Allow the mixture to cool, then mash and mold into 4 burgers. Coat lightly in flour and chill. Broil the burgers on both sides for about 3 minutes and serve, topped with melted Mozzarella and sliced tomato, on burger buns.

Variation
Coat the burgers with wholemeal breadcrumbs, then fry and serve with a tomato or barbecue sauce (see pages 96 and 98).

Garnish chicory; red leaf lettuce; mustard and cress; scallion fleurons (see page 99); celery top; endive

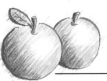

Protein – medium
Fat – low
Fiber – high

Spinach and Blue Cheese Lasagne

½ lb   wholewheat lasagne
1 oz   Parmesan cheese, grated
Mushroom Layers
2 tsp   polyunsaturated oil
2 cups   sliced mushrooms
2 tbsp   wholemeal flour
1 cup   vegetable stock
1 tsp   yeast extract
Spinach and Cheese Layers
¾ lb   fresh spinach
4 tbsp   polyunsaturated margarine
¼ cup   flour
2 cups   low-fat milk
salt and freshly ground pepper
pinch ground nutmeg
2 oz   blue cheese, crumbled

Cook the lasagne in boiling water until tender; drain and refresh in cold water. Meanwhile, heat the oil and sauté the mushrooms just until cooked. Boil the spinach just until cooked; drain off excess water, refresh and chop roughly.

To prepare the sauce for the mushroom layers, mix the flour with a little of the stock to form a smooth paste. Stir in the remaining stock, together with the vegetable extract. Bring to a boil and simmer for 2–3 minutes; add the mushrooms. Cook for 1–2 minutes, then remove from the heat.

To prepare the sauce for the spinach and cheese layers, melt the margarine, add the flour and cook gently for 1–2 minutes. Add the milk gradually and stir the sauce over the heat until thickened. Allow the sauce to cook, then remove from the heat and stir in seasoning and nutmeg. Mix half the sauce with the spinach and blue cheese.

In an ovenproof dish, layer the pasta, mushroom sauce, and spinach and cheese sauce, finishing with a layer of pasta. Pour the remaining sauce over the top and sprinkle with Parmesan cheese. Bake at 400°F for 30 minutes, or until bubbling.

Garnish spinach purée; sliced mushrooms; turned mushroom (see page 99); paprika

Protein – high
Fat – medium
Fiber – high

Egg Bombay

1½ lb	broccoli
5 eggs, hard-boiled	
2 tbsp	mango chutney, chopped
salt and freshly ground pepper	
4 tbsp	polyunsaturated margarine
1 cup	finely chopped onions
1 tbsp	mild curry paste
2 tsp	turmeric
2 tbsp	wholemeal flour
1 cup	low-fat milk
½ cup	plain yogurt
¼ cup	light cream

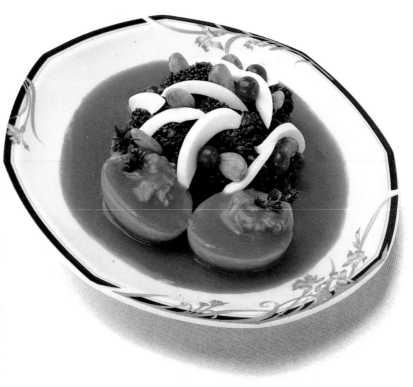

Separate the broccoli into stalks and florets; cook the stalks until tender, then chop finely. Halve the eggs, sieve the yolks and mix with the chopped broccoli stalks, chutney and seasoning. Pipe the mixture into the egg halves, retaining two egg white halves for garnish.

Melt the margarine, add the onions and cook until soft. Add the curry paste and turmeric and cook for 2 minutes. Stir in the flour and cook gently for 1–2 minutes. Gradually add the milk and stir the sauce over the heat until thickened. Allow to cook, then remove from the heat, and stir in the yogurt, cream and seasoning. Place the mixture in a food processor or blender, and blend until smooth.

Meanwhile, cook the broccoli florets until just tender; drain. Arrange the eggs and broccoli in a serving dish and spoon the sauce over the eggs.

Garnish sliced egg white; almonds; red currants; fresh thyme

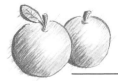

Protein – high
Fat – high
Fiber – medium

Potato Medley

Four 6–8-oz potatoes

Scrub the potatoes well, prick with a fork and bake for about 1 hour at 375°F until soft.

Suggested fillings (for 1 serving)

Pesto: Scoop out the potato flesh, mash with 1 tsp pesto sauce and a little margarine and replace in the potato skin. Mix together 1 tsp grated Parmesan cheese with 1 tsp chopped mixed nuts, sprinkle over the potato and brown under the broiler.

Nutty Cream: Blend together 2 tsp sour cream, 1 tbsp Roquefort cheese, 1 tsp chopped walnuts and a few snipped chives. Scoop out the potato flesh, mash with the cream mixture and replace in the potato skin. Garnish with a walnut half.

Chinese Mushrooms: Scoop out the potato flesh and mash lightly. Stir-fry ¼ cup sliced mushrooms with a dash of soy sauce and place in the potato skin. Top with piped potato and a slice of Mozzarella cheese and brown under the broiler.

Guacamole: Scoop out the potato flesh, mash with a quarter of an avocado, a little margarine, a little cooked crushed garlic (optional), a dash of lemon juice and seasoning. Pipe into the potato skin.

Garnish tomato; Chinese cabbage; fresh thyme; sliced scallion

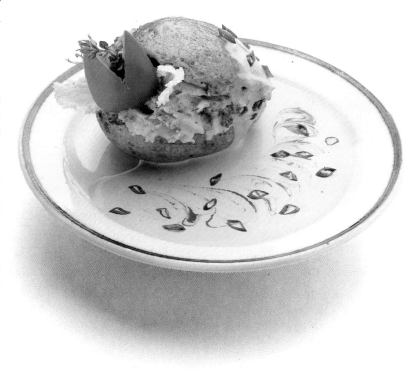

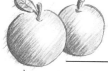

Analysis for Potato only:

Protein – low
Fat – low
Fiber – medium

Dhal

1 cup	lentils
2 tbsp	polyunsaturated oil
1¼ cups	thinly sliced onions
1 tsp	cumin seeds
1 clove garlic, finely chopped	
1 tsp	ground coriander
1 tsp	ground cinnamon
	pinch ground cloves
3 cups	vegetable stock
1 fresh bay leaf	
salt and freshly ground pepper	

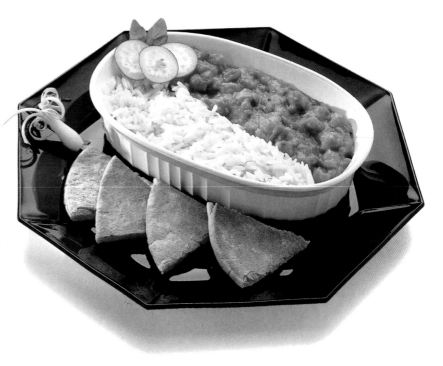

Soak the lentils as required (see page 4). Drain, rinse and place in a pot of cold water. Bring to a boil and cook rapidly for 10 minutes. Drain.

Heat the oil and sauté the onions, cumin seeds and garlic until the onion is soft. Add the coriander and cook for an additional 2–3 minutes.

Stir in the lentils, cinnamon and cloves and cook for 1 minute, stirring constantly. Add the stock, bay leaf and seasoning and bring to a boil. Simmer for 45 minutes. Remove the bay leaf before serving.

Serve with rice or naan bread, accompanied by side dishes such as chutney, fried banana and grated coconut, or serve the dhal as an accompaniment to vegetable curry.

Garnish scallion fleuron (see page 99);
sliced radish; fresh basil

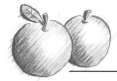

Protein – medium
Fat – medium
Fiber – high

Nutty Hotpot with Cheese Dumplings

1 tbsp   polyunsaturated oil
1/4 lb   onions, cut into wedges
1/4 lb   cauliflower, broken into florets
1/2 cup   peas, fresh or frozen
1/3 cup   green beans
1/2 cup   canned tomatoes, chopped
1/3 cup   sliced zucchini
1 cup   roasted peanuts, unsalted
1 tsp   chopped fresh mixed herbs (oregano, thyme, basil and chives)
1 tsp   yeast extract mixed with 1 1/2 cups   boiling water
Cheese Dumplings
1/2 cup   self-rising wholemeal flour
4 tbsp   polyunsaturated margarine
1 oz   low-fat Cheddar cheese, grated
2 tbsp   rolled oats

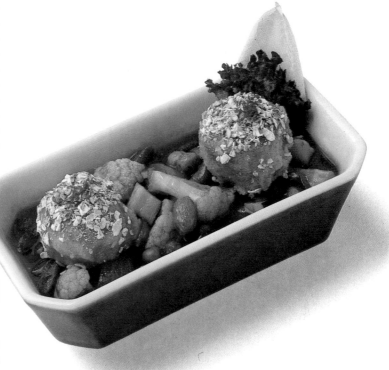

Heat the oil and sauté the onion until soft. Stir in the remaining hotpot ingredients and season well. Cover and simmer for 15 minutes.

Meanwhile, make the dumplings. Sift the flour and rub in the margarine. Mix in the cheese and season well. Add sufficient water to make a soft dough, form into balls and roll lightly in the oats.

Put the hotpot mixture in one large or four individual casseroles. Top with the dumplings and bake at 375°F for 30–40 minutes, until the dumplings are cooked.

Variation
Experiment with seasonal vegetables.

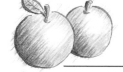

Garnish paprika; chicory; red leaf lettuce

Protein – medium
Fat – high
Fiber – high

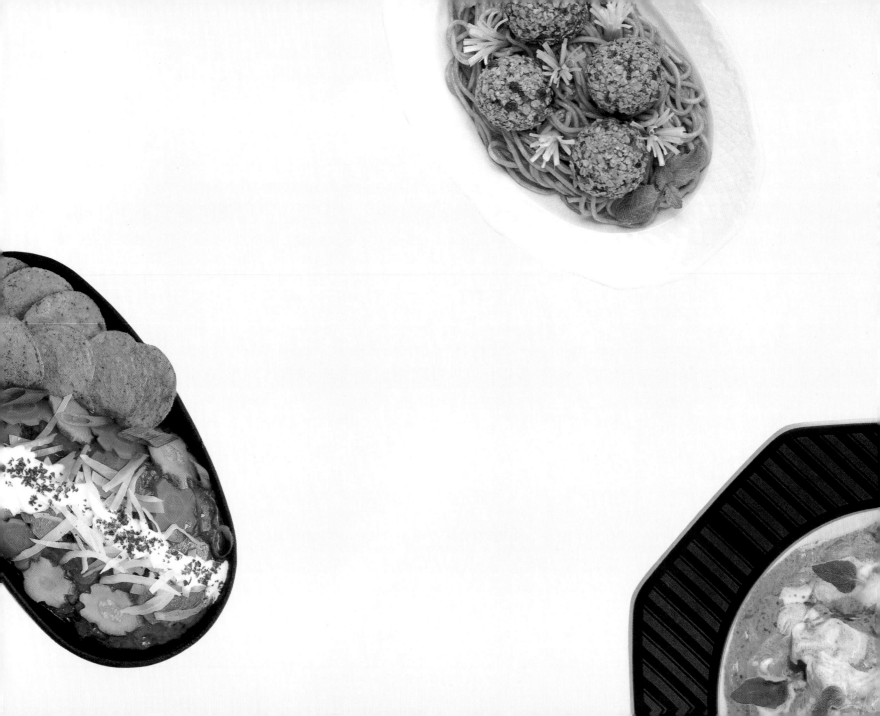

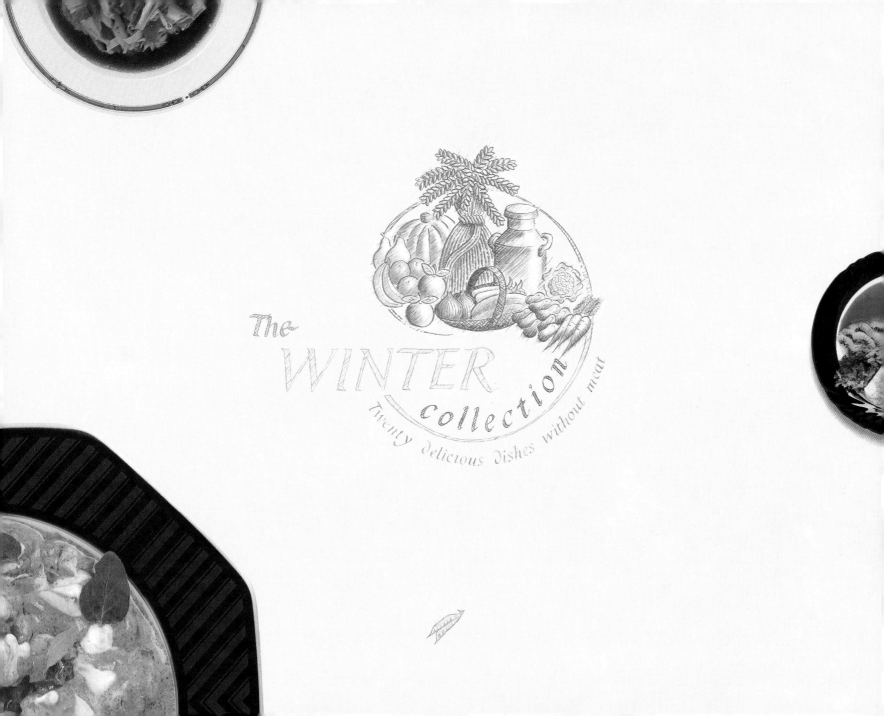

The

WINTER
collection

Twenty delicious dishes without meat

Vegetable Tortilla

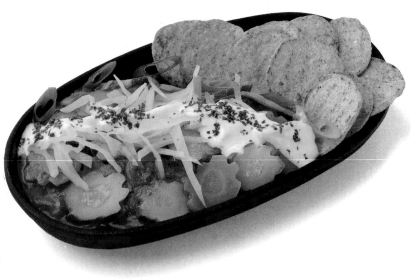

2 tbsp	polyunsaturated oil
1 cup	sliced onions
1 cup	carrots, canelled (see page 102) and sliced
3/4 lb	white cabbage, sliced
3/4 lb	zucchini, canelled (see page 102) and sliced
1 cup	vegetable stock
1/2 cup	tomato juice
2 tbsp	tomato purée
1 tbsp	paprika
1 tsp	chopped fresh mixed herbs (chives, oregano, basil and thyme)
1 tsp	caraway seeds
pinch	ground nutmeg
	salt and freshly ground pepper
2 tbsp	plain yogurt
2 tbsp	light cream
3 oz	tortilla chips

Heat the oil and sauté the onion until soft. Add the carrots, cabbage and zucchini and cook for an additional 5 minutes. Mix thoroughly. Stir in all other ingredients except for the yogurt and cream and simmer for 15–20 minutes.

Transfer the mixture to a serving dish. Mix the yogurt and cream together and pour in a line down the center of the dish.

Serve with tortilla chips.

Variation
Serve with brown rice, noodles, couscous or pita bread instead of the tortilla chips.

Garnish chopped fresh parsley; shredded cabbage; sliced carrots; sliced zucchini; scallion tops cut in diamonds

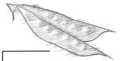

Protein – low
Fat – medium
Fiber – medium

Lemon and Millet Hotpot

½ cup	millet
6 tbsp	polyunsaturated margarine
½ cup	diced onions
1 cup	sliced leeks
½ cup	grated carrots
¼ lb	zucchini, diced
1 stalk celery, diced	
2 tbsp	flour
1 cup	low-fat milk
1 tsp	chopped fresh parsley
1 tsp	chopped fresh sage
grated rind and juice of 1 lemon	
salt and freshly ground pepper	
3 oz	low-fat soft cheese, diced

Cook the millet in boiling water. Melt 4 tbsp of the margarine and sauté the onion, leeks, carrots, zucchini and celery for 10–15 minutes. Add the millet and keep hot.

Meanwhile, melt the remaining margarine, add the flour and cook gently for a few minutes. Add the milk gradually and heat, stirring constantly, to make a smooth sauce. Allow to cook, then stir in the herbs, lemon rind and juice and simmer for 2 minutes. Season. Add 2 oz of the soft cheese and stir over a gentle heat until smooth. Do not allow to boil. Add the vegetables and millet and mix well. Transfer to a serving dish, top with the remaining cheese and brown under the broiler.

Variation
Experiment with seasonal vegetables.

Garnish potato chips; diced red pepper; mustard and cress; fresh rosemary

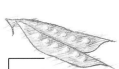

Protein – low
Fat – high
Fiber – medium

Lentil Pilaf

1 tbsp	polyunsaturated oil
½ cup	sliced onions
¾ cup	lentils
1 cup	brown rice
⅓ cup	grated carrots
1 tsp	ground cinnamon
1 tsp	ground cloves
1 tsp	fennel seeds
salt and freshly ground pepper	
2 cups	vegetable stock
½ cup	raisins
½ cup	chopped walnuts

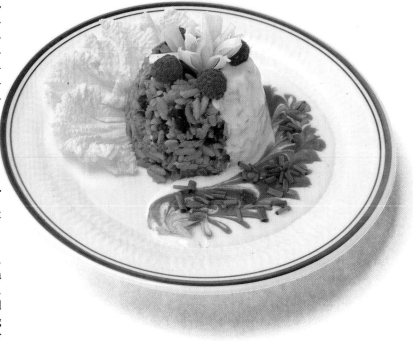

Soak lentils as required (see page 4). Drain, rinse and place in a pot of cold water. Bring to a boil and cook rapidly for 10 minutes. Drain.

Heat the oil and sauté the onion. Stir in the lentils, rice and carrots. Add the cinnamon, cloves, fennel seeds and seasoning and stir over a moderate heat for 2–3 minutes. Add the stock and bring to a boil. Cover, reduce the heat and simmer until the stock is absorbed (about 30 minutes). Stir the mixture to check consistency, adding more water if required. Add the raisins and nuts. Cover and simmer very gently for an additional 10 minutes.

For attractive presentation, press the mixture into a small pudding mold and turn out onto a serving dish. Serve with plain yogurt laced with curry sauce (see page 97).

Variations
Use the pilaf as a stuffing for vegetables, such as squash or peppers, or serve as an accompaniment to another dish.

Replace walnuts with cashews or whole peanuts.

Garnish scallions; Chinese cabbage; raspberries; snipped fresh chives

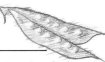

Protein – high
Fat – medium
Fiber – high

Camembert Croquettes

½ lb	*fairly firm Camembert cheese*
2 tbsp	*wholemeal flour*
½ tsp	*dry mustard*
½ tsp	*chopped fresh mixed herbs*
	salt and freshly ground pepper
¼ cup	*wholemeal breadcrumbs*
½ tsp	*chilli powder*
	pinch cayenne pepper
1 egg, beaten	
	polyunsaturated oil
¼ cup	*plain yogurt*

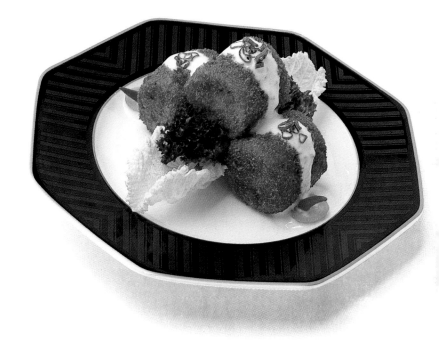

Divide the cheese into 8 portions, wrap in plastic wrap and freeze for 1 hour.

Mix the flour, mustard, herbs and seasoning together, then mix the breadcrumbs with the chilli powder and cayenne. Dip the cheese portions first in the flour mixture, then in the beaten egg and finally in the breadcrumb mixture. Deep-fry the cheese in the oil for about 30 seconds until golden-brown. Drain and serve with a crisp salad and plain yogurt.

Variations
Substitute Brie, Chèvre or Ricotta cheese for the Camembert and vary the coating by mixing oatmeal with breadcrumbs.

Serve this dish with a cranberry sauce or red currant purée.

Garnish plain yogurt; Chinese cabbage;
red leaf lettuce; cherry tomato; red chilli;
sliced scallions

Protein – high
Fat – high
Fiber – low

Vegetable Fusilli

2 tbsp	polyunsaturated margarine
2 tbsp	flour
1 cup	low-fat milk
1/4 lb	low-fat Cheddar cheese, grated
	pinch ground nutmeg
	salt and freshly ground pepper
2/3 cup	sliced mushrooms
1/3 cup	diced mixed sweet peppers
1/3 cup	thinly sliced celery
1/3 cup	thinly sliced zucchini
1/2 lb	wholewheat, egg or spinach fusilli
1/4 cup	peas, fresh or frozen
2 tbsp	Parmesan cheese, grated

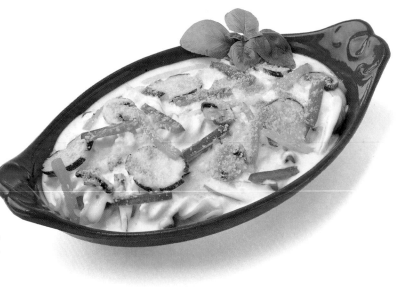

Melt the margarine, add the flour and cook gently for 1–2 minutes. Add the milk gradually and heat, stirring constantly, to obtain a smooth texture. Allow the sauce to cook, then add the grated Cheddar cheese, nutmeg and seasoning.

Sauté the mushrooms, peppers, celery and zucchini lightly, retaining some raw vegetables for the garnish.

Boil the pasta just until cooked. Drain and refresh in cold water.

Combine the cooked vegetables, cheese sauce and pasta with the peas. Turn into an ovenproof dish, sprinkle with Parmesan and bake at 375°F for about 20 minutes, until light brown and bubbling.

Variations
Use different colors and shapes of pasta.

Try different seasonal vegetables.

Garnish blanched vegetables; sprig of fresh basil

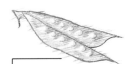

Protein – high
Fat – medium
Fiber – high

Spinach Roulade

1 lb   spinach, chopped
1 bunch watercress, chopped
1 tsp   chopped fresh sage
pinch ground nutmeg
2 tbsp   polyunsaturated margarine
2 tbsp   flour
1 cup   low-fat milk
2 eggs, separated
salt and freshly ground pepper
¾ cup   cream cheese, softened
½ lb   filo pastry
1 egg
2 tbsp   low-fat milk

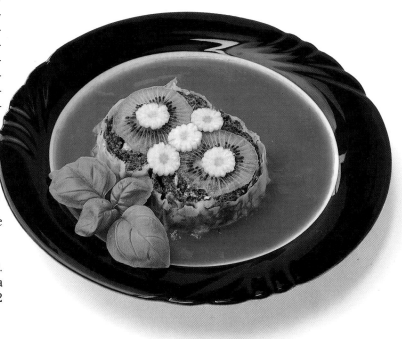

Cook and refresh the spinach. Place in a food processor with the watercress, sage and nutmeg, and blend until smooth.

Melt the margarine, add the flour and cook gently for 1–2 minutes. Gradually add the milk and heat, stirring constantly, to make a smooth sauce. Allow the sauce to cook, then cool slightly. Add the 2 egg yolks and the spinach mixture to the sauce. Mix thoroughly.

Whisk the 2 egg whites to fairly stiff peaks and fold into the sauce. Season. Pour the mixture into a greased and lined jelly roll pan and bake at 350°F for about 20 minutes. Turn out onto wax paper sprinkled lightly with flour and allow to cool. Spread with the cream cheese and roll up like a jelly roll.

Lay one sheet of filo pastry on a clean work surface and brush with cold water. Place a second layer on top and brush with water. Brush all the edges with water and wrap the spinach roll in the pastry, sealing the edges. Combine the egg and milk, and egg wash the pastry. Place the roulade on a greased pan and bake at 400°F until crisp and golden-brown.

Variations

Spread the roulade with a stuffing – such as an apricot and nut combination – before wrapping in the pastry.

Serve the roulade without the pastry cover.

Garnish kiwi fruit slices; baby sweetcorn; fresh basil; tomato sauce (see page 96)

Protein – high
Fat – high
Fiber – low

Winter Cobbler

Filling

¹/₂ lb   eggplant, sliced
¹/₂ cup   chopped onions
¹/₂ cup   sliced carrots
³/₄ lb   zucchini, sliced
³/₄ cup   cauliflower florets
1 cup   canned tomatoes, chopped
1 clove garlic, finely chopped
2 tbsp   tomato purée
dash Tabasco sauce
dash Worcestershire sauce
1 cup   vegetable stock
salt and freshly ground pepper

Topping

¹/₂ cup   wholemeal flour
¹/₂ cup   unbleached flour
2 tsp   baking powder
¹/₂ cup   polyunsaturated margarine
1 cup   low-fat milk

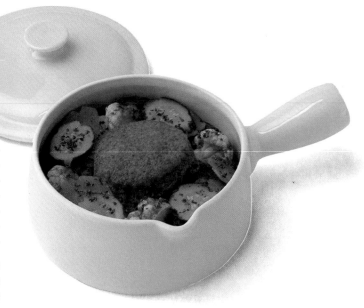

Sprinkle the eggplant slices with salt and allow to drain for 30 minutes, then rinse and dry thoroughly. Carefully combine the ingredients for the filling in a saucepan, reserving some vegetables for garnish, bring to a boil and simmer for 15 minutes.

To prepare the biscuit topping, combine the flours and baking powder, rub in the margarine and add sufficient milk to form a dough. Roll out the dough to a thickness of 1 inch and cut into four 2¼-inch circles.

Put the vegetable mixture in an ovenproof dish and top with the biscuit circles. Bake at 350°F for 20–25 minutes, until the biscuits are puffed and brown. The color can be enhanced by placing under the broiler for a few minutes.

Variations

Boost the protein content by adding cooked lentils to the filling before baking.

For ease of preparation, use a biscuit mix for the topping.

Garnish blanched cauliflower florets; zucchini and carrot slices; chopped fresh parsley

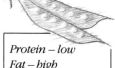

Protein – low
Fat – high
Fiber – medium

Wholemeal Lentil Pancakes

8 pancakes, made with wholemeal flour (see page 16)
Filling
1 cup   lentils
4 tbsp   polyunsaturated margarine
2 tsp   polyunsaturated oil
½ cup   finely chopped onions
1 cup   vegetable stock
1 cup   canned tomatoes, chopped
1 tsp   ground coriander
1 tsp   tomato purée
½ tsp   brown sugar
2 tbsp   red wine (optional)
1½ cups   sliced mushrooms
Parsley Sauce
2 tbsp   polyunsaturated margarine
2 tbsp   flour
1 cup   low-fat milk
¼ cup   plain yogurt
2 tsp   chopped fresh parsley
½ tsp   lemon juice
salt and freshly ground pepper

Soak the lentils as required (see page 4). Drain, rinse and place in a pot of cold water. Bring to a boil and cook rapidly for 10 minutes. Drain.

To make the filling, heat the margarine and oil together and sauté the onion until soft. Add the lentils, stock, tomatoes, coriander, tomato purée, sugar and wine and simmer gently, uncovered, for about 30 minutes. Add the mushrooms and cook for 5 minutes.

To make the sauce, melt the margarine, add the flour and cook for 1–2 minutes. Add the milk gradually and stir over a gentle heat to make a smooth sauce. Add the remaining ingredients and cook gently for a few minutes.

Fill each pancake with the lentil mixture, roll or fold and arrange in a dish. Blanket with parsley sauce and serve piping hot.

Garnish diced red pepper; sliced kiwi fruit; red leaf lettuce; chicory leaves; fresh thyme

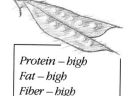

Protein – high
Fat – high
Fiber – high

Cashew and Mushroom Loaf

1 tbsp   polyunsaturated oil
1/2 cup   finely chopped onions
1 clove garlic, finely chopped
1 1/4 cups   cashew nuts
1/3 cup   fresh wholemeal breadcrumbs
1 egg, beaten
2 medium parsnips, cooked and mashed
1 tsp   fresh rosemary, chopped
1 tsp   fresh thyme, chopped
1 tsp   yeast extract
1/2 cup   hot vegetable stock
salt and freshly ground pepper
1 tbsp   polyunsaturated margarine
1 1/2 cups   sliced mushrooms

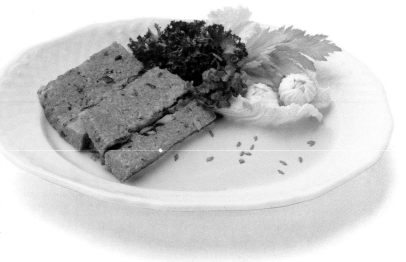

Heat the oil and sauté the onion and garlic until soft. Grind the cashew nuts in a blender and mix with the breadcrumbs. Add the egg and mix in the mashed parsnips and herbs. Add the onion and garlic. Dissolve the yeast extract in the hot stock and add to the other ingredients. Season well. Adjust consistency with stock or breadcrumbs. Melt the margarine and sauté the mushrooms.

Grease a 1-lb loaf pan and press in half the nut mixture, then cover with a layer of mushrooms and top with the rest of the nut mixture. Cover with foil and bake at 350°F for 1 hour. Let stand for 10 minutes, then turn out. The loaf may be served hot or cold.

Variations
Use wild mushrooms for an unusual but more expensive combination.

Substitute asparagus for the mushrooms.

Garnish dressing made by combining plain yogurt with a little tomato purée and honey to flavor; red leaf lettuce; turned mushrooms (see page 99); celery tops; Chinese cabbage; mustard and cress

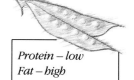

Protein – low
Fat – high
Fiber – low

Chinese Vegetables with Pasta

½ lb   wholewheat noodles or tagliatelle
½ cup   carrots, canelled (see page 102) and sliced
½ cup   turnips, cut in julienne strips
½ cup   daikon radish, canelled (see page 102) and sliced
½ cup   celery, sliced at an angle
½ cup   red and green peppers, cut in diamonds
⅓ cup   green beans, cut in 1-inch lengths
⅓ cup   beansprouts
½ cup   pineapple juice
2 tbsp   soy sauce
small piece of fresh ginger, peeled and chopped
salt and freshly ground pepper
2 tbsp   polyunsaturated oil
2 tbsp   polyunsaturated margarine
1¼ cups   sliced mushrooms

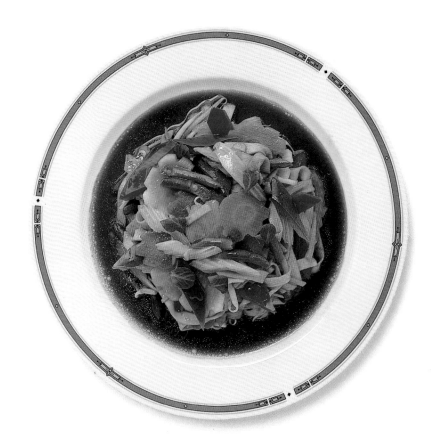

Cook the noodles in boiling, salted water until just cooked. Drain and refresh in cold water. Blanch the carrots, turnips, daikon radish, celery, peppers and green beans in boiling water for 4 minutes. Refresh and drain. Retain some vegetables for garnish. Rinse and drain the beansprouts. Blend the pineapple juice with ½ cup cold water and the soy sauce, ginger and seasoning. Set aside.

Heat the oil and margarine together in a large pan or wok and stir-fry all the vegetables, except the mushrooms and beansprouts, for 3 minutes. Add the pineapple juice mixture and stir-fry for an additional 5 minutes. Stir in the noodles, mushrooms and beansprouts and fry for 2 minutes. Serve immediately.

Variation
Increase the protein content by adding cooked lentils to the mixture.

Garnish blanched vegetables; fresh basil

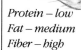

Protein – low
Fat – medium
Fiber – high

Walnut and Roquefort Savory

2 tbsp	polyunsaturated margarine
1/3 cup	finely chopped onions
3/4 lb	potatoes
2 tsp	chopped fresh parsley
1 tbsp	skimmed milk powder
	pinch ground nutmeg
	salt and freshly ground pepper
	3 egg whites, stiffly beaten
1/2 lb	blue cheese (Stilton, Roquefort or Danish Blue)
4 oz	cottage cheese
	3 egg yolks
1/2 cup	plain yogurt
3/4 cup	walnut halves

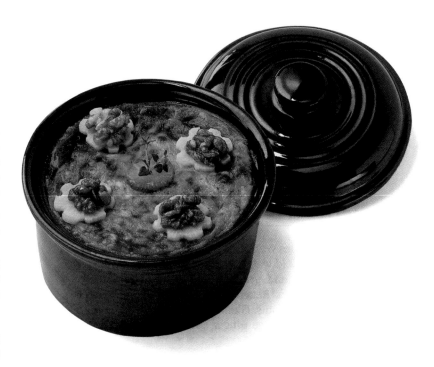

Melt the margarine and sauté the onions until soft; drain off the margarine and reserve. Boil and drain the potatoes, reserving the cooking water. Mash the potatoes and stir in the onion and parsley. Add the reserved margarine, milk powder, nutmeg and seasoning and enough of the potato water to make a light mixture. Beat the mixture well. Fold in the egg whites carefully and put the mixture in a well-greased ovenproof dish.

Mix the cheeses together, add the egg yolks and yogurt and mix thoroughly. Pour this mixture over the potatoes and garnish with the walnut halves.

Bake at 350°F for 30 minutes until the top is golden-brown. Serve accompanied by a crisp salad.

Garnish sliced strawberry; fresh thyme;
sliced daikon radish; walnut halves

Protein – high
Fat – high
Fiber – low

Chilli Beans

⅔ cup	dried mixed beans

(borlotti, cannellini and haricot, shown in the photograph)

1 tbsp	polyunsaturated oil
½ cup	chopped onions
Chilli Sauce	
2 tbsp	soft brown sugar
2 tbsp	soy sauce
2 tbsp	wine vinegar
1 tsp	tomato purée
1 tsp	dry mustard
½ tsp	chilli powder
1 tsp	paprika
1 cup	vegetable stock
½ cup	sliced red peppers
1 tsp	potato flour (fecule)

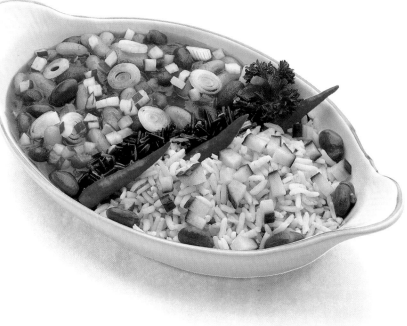

Soak the beans overnight (see page 3). Drain, rinse and place in separate pots of cold water. Bring to a boil and cook rapidly for 10 minutes. Reduce the heat and simmer for required time. Drain. Alternatively use 2 cups canned or cooked mixed beans.

Heat the oil and sauté the onion until soft. Combine all the sauce ingredients except the stock, peppers and potato flour and add to the onion. Cook for 5 minutes, then add the stock, red peppers and beans. Bring to a boil and simmer for 10 minutes.

Blend the potato flour with a little cold water, add to the mixture and stir until thickened. Serve with brown and wild rice or wholewheat pasta.

Garnish red chillis; diced cucumber; diced radish; sliced scallion

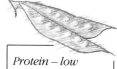

Protein – low
Fat – low
Fiber – high

Cheese and Vegetable Macaroni

6 oz	wholewheat or egg macaroni
4 tbsp	polyunsaturated margarine
2 cups	chopped leeks
1/4 cup	flour
3 cups	low-fat milk
1/2 lb	low-fat Cheddar cheese, grated
	salt and freshly ground pepper
1/4 cup	wholemeal breadcrumbs
1 tsp	snipped fresh chives

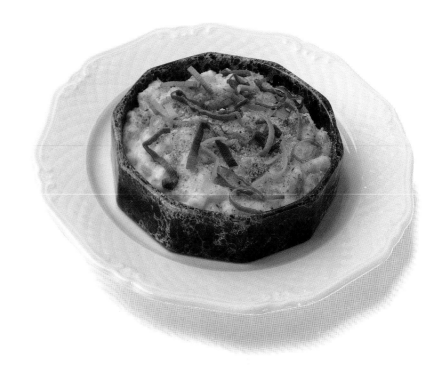

Cook the macaroni until just tender. Drain well and refresh in cold water. Melt the margarine and sauté the leeks for 2 minutes. Stir in the flour and cook for a minute. Gradually stir in the milk and heat, stirring constantly, to make a smooth sauce. Add three-quarters of the cheese and all the macaroni and season well.

Spoon the mixture into an ovenproof dish. Combine the bread-crumbs, chives and remaining cheese and sprinkle evenly over the top of the dish. Bake at 375°F for 30–35 minutes, until golden-brown.

Variations
Try other seasonal vegetables.

Use pasta shapes instead of macaroni.

Mix sesame seeds with the cheese topping to
vary the flavor.

Garnish julienne of leeks, blanched

Protein – high
Fat – high
Fiber – high

Lentil Turnovers

³⁄₄ cup   lentils
¹⁄₂ lb   rutabagas, diced
2 cups   vegetable stock
1 fresh bay leaf
salt and freshly ground pepper
2 tbsp   polyunsaturated margarine
¹⁄₂ cup   finely chopped onions
2 tsp   chopped fresh mixed herbs (basil, chives, oregano and thyme)
1 tbsp   tomato purée
¹⁄₂ lb   puff pastry
¹⁄₄ lb   Mozzarella cheese, sliced
1 egg
2 tbsp   low-fat milk

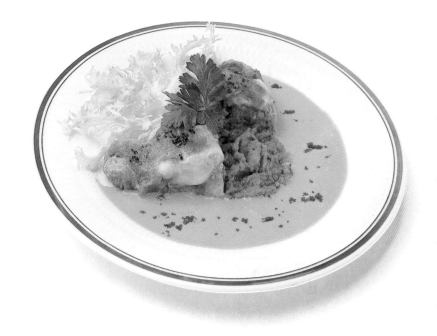

Soak lentils as required (see page 4). Drain, rinse and place in a pot of cold water. Bring to a boil and cook rapidly for 10 minutes. Drain.

Cook, drain and mash the rutabagas. Meanwhile, place the lentils, stock, bay leaf and seasoning in a pot and simmer for 30 minutes until the lentils are tender. Drain if necessary and remove the bay leaf. Melt the margarine and sauté the onion until golden. Mix in the rutabagas and lentils and add the herbs and tomato purée.

Roll out the pastry dough and cut into four 6-inch circles. Spoon a portion of the lentil mixture onto half of each circle. Brush the pastry edges with water, then fold over and press the edges together firmly to seal. Place the turnovers on an oiled baking pan. Mix the egg and milk, and use to brush the turnovers. Top with Mozzarella slices and bake at 425°F for 15 minutes.

Serve with lentil Béchamel (see page 96).

Garnish endive; flat-leaf parsley; paprika

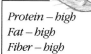

Protein – high
Fat – high
Fiber – high

Vegetable Symphony

1 medium head cauliflower, broken into florets
1 lb zucchini, canelled (see page 102) and sliced
1¼ cups sliced mushrooms
4 tbsp polyunsaturated margarine
2 tbsp flour
1 cup low-fat milk
salt and freshly ground pepper
¼ lb low-fat soft cheese
1 tbsp wholemeal breadcrumbs
1 tbsp pine nuts
1 tsp snipped fresh chives

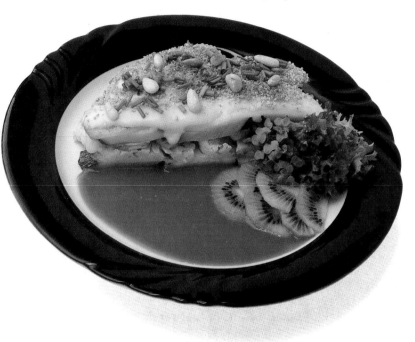

Cook the cauliflower and zucchini in separate pots of boiling water until just tender; drain. Meanwhile, cook the mushrooms in half the margarine for 3–4 minutes; drain.

Layer half the zucchini, all the cauliflower and all the mushrooms in an ovenproof dish; top with remaining zucchini. Melt the remaining margarine, add the flour and cook for 1–2 minutes. Stir in the milk and continue stirring until the sauce thickens. Allow to cook, then season and add the cheese. Pour the sauce over the vegetables and sprinkle the top with breadcrumbs. Place under the broiler until lightly browned. Sprinkle with pine nuts and snipped chives before serving.

Serve accompanied by a tomato sauce (see page 96).

Garnish kiwi fruit; red leaf lettuce; cress

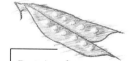

Protein – low
Fat – medium
Fiber – low

Midwinter Pie

2 lb potatoes, cooked
½ cup low-fat milk
2 tbsp polyunsaturated margarine
pinch ground nutmeg
1 egg
1¼ cups sliced onions
1¼ cups broccoli florets
¼ cup wholemeal breadcrumbs
1 tsp chopped fresh rosemary
1 tsp chopped fresh parsley
1 tsp chopped fresh basil
2 oz Parmesan cheese, grated
salt and freshly ground pepper
¼ lb low-fat Cheddar cheese, grated

Mash or whip half the potatoes with the milk, margarine, nutmeg and egg or, as an alternative, separate the eggs, add the yolks to the potato mixture, then whip the whites stiffly and fold into the potato purée. Cut the remaining potatoes into slices. Sauté the onions in a little margarine but do not allow to turn brown.

Steam or boil the broccoli until tender but still crisp. Meanwhile, mix the breadcrumbs, herbs, Parmesan and seasoning. Cover the bottom of an oiled casserole with the sliced potatoes. Follow with the onions, Cheddar cheese and broccoli. Top with the mashed potato mixture and sprinkle with the breadcrumb mixture. Bake at 375°F for about 15 minutes until lightly browned.

Serve accompanied by Béchamel and yogurt sauce (see page 96).

Variation
Replace the broccoli with another vegetable, such as leek or cauliflower.

Garnish sliced strawberry; watercress

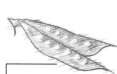

Protein – high
Fat – medium
Fiber – high

Nutty Vegetable Flan

½ lb	wholemeal pastry
1 cup	cauliflower florets
½ cup	chopped carrots
½ cup	diced green beans
½ green pepper, diced	
½ cup	roasted peanuts
2 eggs	
1 cup	low-fat milk
2 oz	Edam cheese, grated
salt and freshly ground pepper	

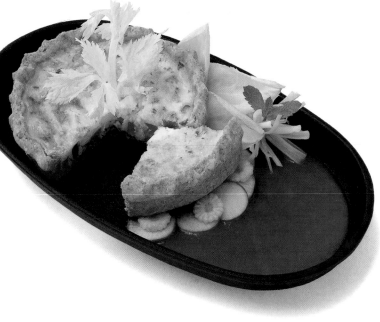

Line 1 large or 4 small flan dishes with the pastry and bake blind (see page 102).

Blanch all the vegetables, refresh in cold water and divide among the pastry cases. Roughly chop the peanuts and sprinkle evenly over the vegetables. Beat the eggs and milk together. Mix in the cheese, season and pour the mixture over the vegetables.

Bake the flan at 350°F for about 25 minutes, until the filling is set. Serve hot or cold accompanied by tomato sauce (see page 96).

Variation
Experiment with different vegetables and nuts.

Garnish chicory leaves; scallion fleuron (see page 99); mint leaf; celery top; sliced radish; baby sweetcorn

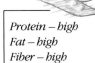

Protein – high
Fat – high
Fiber – high

Fresh Herb Oatcakes

1 tbsp	polyunsaturated oil
1/2 cup	finely chopped onions
5 oz	low-fat Cheddar cheese, finely grated
1/2 cup	wholemeal breadcrumbs
1/2 tsp	chopped fresh thyme
1/2 tsp	chopped fresh rosemary
1/2 tsp	chopped fresh sage
	pinch ground nutmeg
	pinch dry mustard
	salt and freshly ground pepper
1 egg, beaten	
1 egg	
2 tbsp	low-fat milk
2 tbsp	rolled oats

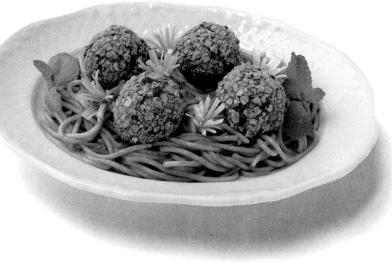

Heat the oil and sauté the onion until soft. Allow to cool. Mix the onion with the cheese, breadcrumbs, herbs, nutmeg, mustard and seasonings. Combine with the beaten egg. Shape the mixture into balls. Whisk the egg and milk lightly. Dip the balls in the egg wash and coat with the rolled oats. Shallow-fry until lightly browned and then bake at 425°F for 15–20 minutes.

Serve with a dip, such as garlic mayonnaise, or to make a more substantial dish, serve with wholewheat spaghetti in a curry sauce (see page 97), as shown.

Garnish mint leaves; scallion fleuron (see page 99)

Protein – high
Fat – medium
Fiber – low

Indonesian-style Vegetables

2 tbsp   polyunsaturated oil
$^1/_2$ cup   chopped onions
1 clove garlic, finely chopped
$^1/_2$ tsp   turmeric
$^1/_2$ tsp   paprika
$^1/_2$ tsp   ground cumin
$^1/_2$ tsp   dry mustard
2 tbsp   tomato purée
$^1/_2$ vegetable stock cube
1 lb   potatoes, cut into 1-inch cubes
1 head cauliflower, broken into florets
$1^1/_2$ cups   water
salt and freshly ground pepper
small piece fresh ginger, peeled and finely chopped
$^1/_2$ cup   plain yogurt
$^1/_2$ tsp   chopped fresh coriander
$^1/_2$ tsp   chopped fresh mint

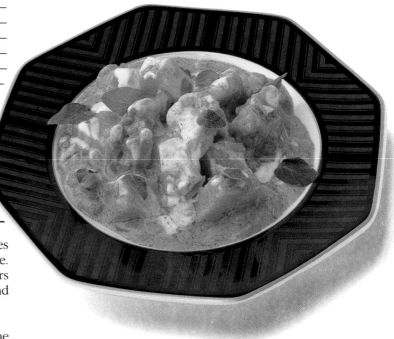

Heat the oil and sauté the onion and garlic until soft. Add the spices and stir well. Stir in the tomato purée and the crumbled stock cube. Add the potatoes and cauliflower, stirring well so that the flavors blend. Add the water, seasoning and ginger. Bring to a boil and simmer for 15–20 minutes, until all the vegetables are just cooked.

Strain off a little of the cooking liquid into a bowl and blend in the yogurt. Stir this mixture into the vegetables. Mix well, sprinkle with the chopped herbs and serve with wholewheat pasta shells, macaroni or brown rice.

Variation
To increase the protein content, add sliced hard-boiled eggs or cooked chickpeas.

Garnish fresh oregano leaves; plain yogurt

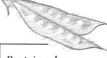

Protein – low
Fat – medium
Fiber – medium

Beanfeast

²/₃ cup	*dried mixed beans*
¹/₄ cup	*dried green split peas*
4 tbsp	*polyunsaturated margarine*
1 tbsp	*polyunsaturated oil*
	2 leeks, chopped
	2 carrots, chopped
	2 stalks celery, chopped
	1 onion, sliced
	2 zucchini, sliced
¹/₂ cup	*canned tomatoes, chopped*
²/₃ cup	*sliced mushrooms*
1 tbsp	*fine oatmeal*
2 tbsp	*tomato purée*
2¹/₂ cups	*vegetable stock*
2 tsp	*yeast extract*
¹/₂ tsp	*ground mace*
¹/₂ tsp	*chopped fresh mint*
¹/₂ tsp	*ground coriander*
1 tsp	*chopped parsley*
1 tsp	*chopped fresh thyme*

Parsley Dumplings

4 tbsp	*polyunsaturated margarine*
¹/₂ cup	*self-rising wholemeal flour*
2 tsp	*chopped fresh parsley*

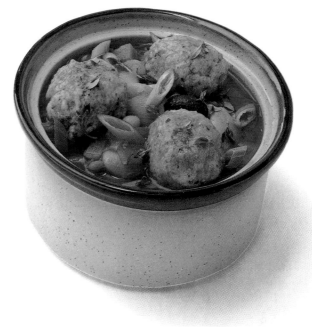

Soak the beans and peas overnight (see page 3). Drain, and place in separate pots of cold water. Bring to a boil and cook rapidly for 10 minutes. Reduce heat and simmer for required time. Drain. Alternatively use 2 cups canned or cooked mixed beans and ½ cup canned or cooked green split peas.

Heat the margarine and oil together and sauté the vegetables for 15 minutes. Stir in the oatmeal and cook for 1 minute, then add the beans, tomato purée and stock, and cook for an additional 20 minutes.

To make the dumplings: rub the margarine into the flour, then add the parsley and enough cold water to mix to a soft dough. Divide the dough into four dumplings, and steam, covered, over a pan of boiling water for 15 minutes. Add the yeast extract, mace and herbs to the bean mixture. Place the dumplings on top and simmer, covered, for about 20 minutes.

Garnish chopped scallions; fresh thyme

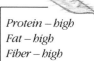

Protein – *high*
Fat – *high*
Fiber – *high*

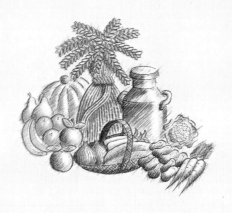

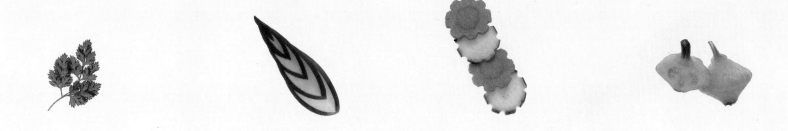 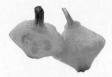

Sauces, Garnishes and Sandwiches

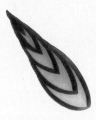 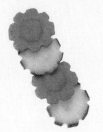

Sauce Recipes

These appetizing sauces have been adapted to reflect the trend for healthy eating. Provided the ingredients are used in the given quantities, each sauce contains less fat than the traditional recipe. The sauces can be served with any appropriate dish in addition to the suggestions made in the seasonal recipes.

White Béchamel Sauce
Makes about 2 cups

4 tbsp   polyunsaturated margarine
¼ cup   flour
2 cups   low-fat milk
1 onion clouté (see page 102)

Heat the milk with the onion until just below boiling point. Remove from the heat and allow to stand for 15 minutes.

Melt the margarine, stir in the flour and cook for a few minutes over a gentle heat without allowing the roux to change color. Remove from the heat and allow to cool.

Strain the milk and add to the roux gradually to make a smooth sauce. Heat, stirring until smooth, replace the onion and allow to cook.

Remove the onion, season to taste and strain if necessary.

Variations
YOGURT   Replace ½ cup of the low-fat milk with plain yogurt, adding it after the sauce has been made. Do not allow the sauce to boil after adding the yogurt.

CHEESE   Add 2 oz grated low-fat Cheddar cheese to the Béchamel sauce, remove from the heat and do not allow to boil.

ONION   Sauté ½ cup chopped or diced onions in polyunsaturated margarine until soft, not allowing the onions to change color. Add to the Béchamel sauce.

MUSHROOM   Sauté 1¼ cups well-washed, sliced white button mushrooms without allowing them to change color, add to the sauce and simmer for 10 minutes.

SPINACH   Process the Béchamel sauce in a blender or food processor with ½ cup cooked chopped spinach flavored with a pinch of nutmeg.

LENTIL   Add a purée of ¼ cup lentils – soaked, cooked and drained – to the basic Béchamel sauce.

MINT   Add freshly chopped mint to the basic Béchamel sauce.

Tomato Sauce
Makes about 1 cup

1 tbsp   polyunsaturated margarine
⅓ cup   chopped onion
⅓ cup   chopped carrot
3 tbsp   chopped celery
½ bay leaf
sprig of thyme
1 tbsp   wholemeal flour
¼ cup   tomato purée
1½ cups   vegetable stock, boiling
salt and freshly ground pepper

Melt the margarine. Add the onion, carrot, celery, bay leaf and thyme, and brown slightly. Blend in the flour and cook to a sandy texture, allowing the mixture to change color slightly. Stir in the tomato purée and allow to cool. Add the boiling stock gradually and again bring to a boil, stirring constantly. Season and allow to simmer for 1 hour.

Adjust the seasoning and either process or pass through a sieve.

"Quick" Tomato Sauce
Makes about 1 cup

2 tbsp   polyunsaturated margarine
$^1/_3$ cup   finely chopped onion
1 cup   vegetable stock
2 cups   canned tomatoes, chopped
1 clove garlic, finely chopped
1 tbsp   tomato purée
1 tsp   chopped fresh basil
salt and freshly ground pepper

Melt the margarine and sauté the onion until soft. Add the remaining ingredients, bring to a boil, stirring, then simmer, uncovered, for 20 minutes. Adjust the seasoning and either purée in a blender or food processor or pass through a sieve.

Variation
Make a spicy tomato sauce by adding a few drops of Worcestershire sauce and a litte chilli to taste.

Curry Sauce
Makes about 1 cup

2 tbsp   polyunsaturated margarine
$^1/_3$ cup   finely chopped onion
$^1/_2$ clove garlic, finely chopped
1 tbsp   wholemeal flour
2 tsp   curry powder
2 tsp   tomato purée
1$^1/_2$ cups   vegetable stock, boiling
$^1/_4$ cup   chopped apple
2 tsp   dried coconut
1 tsp   sultanas
1 tsp   chopped chutney
2 tsp   ground ginger
salt and freshly ground pepper

Melt the margarine and sauté the onion and garlic without allowing them to change color. Blend in the flour and curry powder and cook to a sandy texture. Stir in the tomato purée. Add the boiling stock gradually, stirring constantly to make a smooth sauce. Add the remaining ingredients and allow the sauce to simmer for 30 minutes. Adjust the seasoning.

For a smooth sauce, either purée in a blender or food processor or pass through a sieve.

Barbecue Sauce
Makes about 1 cup

1 tbsp	polyunsaturated oil
1/3 cup	finely chopped onion
1 clove garlic, finely chopped	
1/2 tsp	dry mustard
1 tbsp	Worcestershire sauce
2 tbsp	malt vinegar
1 tbsp	tomato purée
2 tbsp	light brown sugar
1/2 tsp	chilli seasoning
3/4 cup	vegetable stock

Heat the oil and sauté the onion and garlic until soft. Stir in the mustard, Worcestershire sauce, vinegar, tomato purée, sugar, chilli seasoning and vegetable stock. Bring to a boil, cover and simmer for 7–8 minutes until slightly thickened.

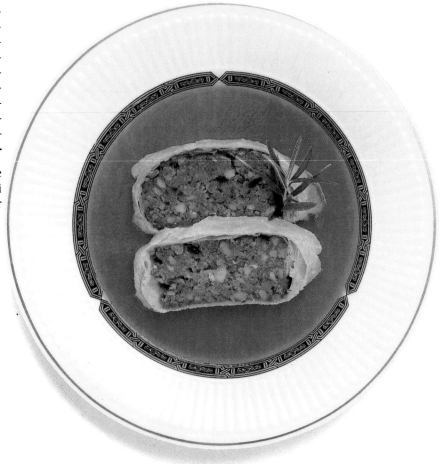

Garnishes for Different Seasons

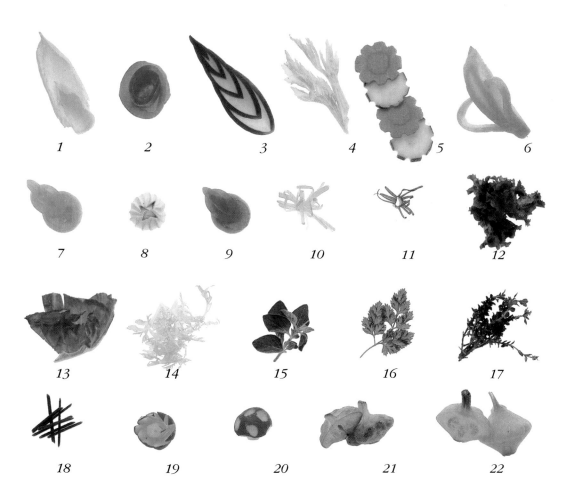

The garnishes shown in the photographs are only suggestions. They can be interchanged according to the season and availability.

1   Chicory
2   Tomato Rose
3   Feathered Apple
4   Celery Top
5   Canelled Carrot and Zucchini
6   Kenley-style Lemon
7   Feathered Yellow Cherry Tomato
8   Turned Button Mushroom
9   Feathered Red Cherry Tomato
10 Scallion Fleuron
11 Scallion Top
12 Red Leaf Lettuce
13 Radicchio
14 Spider Endive
15 Oregano
16 Dill
17 Thyme
18 Chives
19 Radish Rose
20 Toadstool Radish
21 Green Patty Pan Squash
22 Yellow Patty Pan Squash

Vegetarian Sandwiches

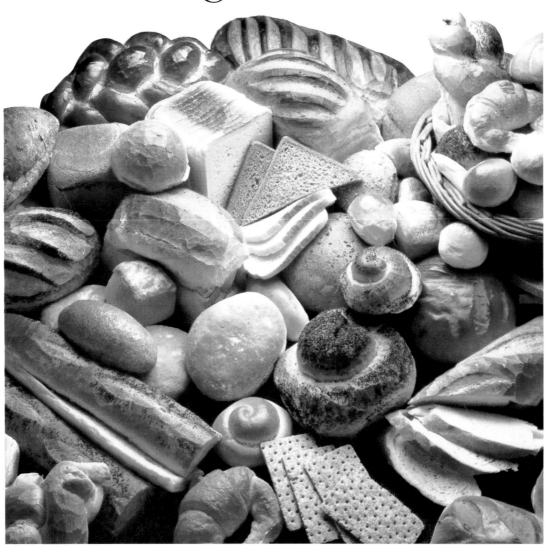

Types of Bread

Choose from the large range of breads that are now widely available to make imaginative sandwiches. Rolls can also be used.

Wholewheat
Wheatgerm
Rye Bread
Raisin Bread
Chapattis/Naan Bread
Malt Bread
Muffins
Sesame Bread

Wholemeal
Multi Grain
Soft Rye
Cheese Bread
Soda Bread
Pita Bread/Tacos
Pumpernickel
French Bread
Croissants
Bagels

30 Suggestions for fillings

Cream cheese, diced celery and roasted peanuts

Grated cheese, beansprouts and dash of soy sauce

Honey, mashed banana and a sprinkling of dried coconut

Cottage cheese mixed with diced apricot on Chinese cabbage

Dates cooked in lemon juice and water, mashed and chilled; spread thickly, top with cream cheese and chopped nuts

Edam cheese and sliced apples, topped with a fruit chutney

Sesame paste topped with beansprouts and sprinkled with sultanas

Peanut butter and yeast extract

Sliced avocado, topped with tomato, mayonnaise and a sprinkling of sunflower seeds

Cooked beans, lightly mashed with chicory leaves and sliced cucumber

Hummus, shredded lettuce and grated carrot

Thinly sliced nut roast and chutney

Diced Feta cheese and finely diced apple mixed with coleslaw

Chopped radish and red or green peppers mixed with cream cheese, topped with endive

Cold lentil dahl topped with tomato and a little yogurt dressing

Cottage cheese mixed with chopped avocado and cashew nuts

Mashed banana mixed with chopped dates and chopped mixed nuts

Chinese cabbage topped with a potato and chive salad

Crunchy peanut butter topped with sliced banana and apple and sprinkled with lemon juice to preserve the color

Yeast extract topped with cornflakes

Cream cheese topped with sliced mushrooms and beansprouts

Chopped Brie, mixed with diced apple, celery and cashew nuts – combine with a light yogurt dressing

Thinly sliced Stilton cheese topped with sliced pear and endive

Crème fraîche topped with a muesli mixture and slices of apple

Cream cheese flavored with pesto sauce topped with tomato slices

Sliced vegetable pâté topped with relish and shredded lettuce

Apricot jam, banana slices and flaked almonds

Shredded white cabbage, chopped red or green peppers and tomato in a sour cream dressing, piled on a bed of watercress

Mushroom pâté spread with a wholegrain mustard

Chilled, cooked and puréed chickpeas, mixed with diced mixed red and green peppers, topped with Chinese cabbage

Glossary of Terms

Definitions of some possibly unfamiliar terms used in the recipes in this book.

BAKE BLIND Place a sheet of wax paper in the lined flan ring and fill with raw haricot beans. Bake at 400°F for about 15 minutes. Remove the beans and paper and bake the flan in the oven for an additional 10 minutes.

BECHAMEL A basic white sauce prepared by gradually adding heated milk to a white roux (cooked without allowing to change color). The sauce is stirred over a gentle heat until it thickens, and then allowed to cook.

BLANCH Food (usually vegetables) is lowered into boiling water and quickly removed. Blanching helps to preserve color and texture.

BUCKWHEAT FLOUR A strong flour with a distinctive flavor made from buckwheat grain. It is advisable to mix it with a white flour to lighten the texture.

BULGUR WHEAT Also known as cracked wheat. Soak for 30 minutes, drain and cover with two parts cold water to one of bulgur. Bring to a boil and simmer for 10–15 minutes. Serve hot as an accompaniment to curries, cold with salads, or as a substitute for rice.

CANELLE A knife with a special groove for channelling fruit or vegetables. See the garnishes on page 99 for an example.

CHAYOTE A pear-shaped vegetable of the squash family. The chayote's skin and almond-shaped seed should be removed before the vegetable is boiled, sautéed, baked, broiled, or fried.

COULIS A term for a smooth sauce or liquid purée which can be sweet (eg: raspberry) or savory (eg: tomato).

COUSCOUS A cereal processed from semolina. It is usually steamed for about 1 hour. Serve as an accompaniment to main course dishes.

DARIOLE MOLD A rounded metal container with a flat base, about the size of a cup. Used for mousses and other mixtures which are turned out before serving.

MILLET Probably the first cereal grain to be used for domestic purposes. It is richer in vitamins, mineral and fat content than other grains. Use as an unusual alternative to rice.

OKRA A pod-like vegetable which can act as a thickening agent in some dishes. To prepare, wash and cut off the thick end. Okra can be deep-fried, microwaved, stewed, boiled or steamed.

ONION CLOUTE An onion studded with 4 cloves and one bay leaf. Infuse in milk to add flavor to sauces.

REFRESH

Literally "to cool down," the term is applied especially to cooked vegetables. They are immediately plunged into ice cold water to cool as quickly as possible.

RICOTTA

A low-fat soft cheese made from whey that is suitable for vegetarians.

ROUX

A thickening element in sauces, made from equal quantities of flour and melted margarine. The mixture is stirred over a gentle heat to cook. The darker the required sauce, the longer the roux is cooked.

SCALLION FLEURON

Cut the top of a scallion into thin strips to three-quarters of the length of the stem, leaving the base attached. Put in iced water until the strips have curled.

SESAME SEEDS

From the sesame plant, the seeds are rich in vitamins and minerals. Used to make tahini (sesame paste).

TOFU

A pale-colored, fermented soy bean curd of light texture, slightly thicker than cottage cheese. Delicious served in a well-flavored sauce or dip.

WILD RICE

Quite different in taste from other types of rice, a traditional accompaniment to some classic dishes. Also effective mixed with long-grain rice to enhance its texture and appearance.

Index

Aduki beans 3

Bake blind, to 102
Baked beans – see haricot beans
Baked Broccoli with Tomato 17
Barbecue Sauce 98
Batter mixture 8
Beanfeast 93
Beans 2
    cooking of 3
Beans, mixed
    Beanfeast 93
    Chilli Beans 85
    Harvest Burgers 66
Béchamel 102
Black beans 3
Black-eyed peas 3
Blanch, to 102
Bread, types of 100
Bread basket, for garnish 5
Broad beans 3
Broccoli, baked with Tomato 17
Buckwheat flour 102
Bulgur wheat 102
Butter beans 3
    Butter Bean Kiev 56
    Lima Bean Curry 34
    Wholesome Hotpot 26
Butter Bean Kiev 56

Camembert Croquettes 77
Canelle, to 102
Canellini beans 4
Canneloni Verdi 15
Capsicum and Chickpea Couscous 35

Cashew and Mushroom Loaf 82
Cashew Paella 9
Cauliflower
    Hot Crudité! 8
    Indonesian-style Vegetables 92
    Lentil and Cauliflower Spice 23
    Pasta del Bria 47
    Summer Vegetables with Wild Rice 42
    Vegetable Symphony 88
Chayote 102
    Chayote Almondine 36
    Ratatouille 32
Cheddar Roast 40
Cheese
    Camembert Croquettes 77
    Cheddar Roast 40
    Cheese Dumplings 71
    Cheese and Vegetable Macaroni 86
    "Crisp" Savory Cheesecake 43
    Eggplant Layer 49
    Pasta del Bria 47
    Vegetable Cheesecake 21
    Walnut and Roquefort Savory 84
    Zucchini Crunch 48
    – see also Fillings for sandwiches
Cheese and Vegetable Macaroni 86
Chickpeas 4
    Capsicum and Chickpea Couscous 35
    Chickpeas Provençale 20
    Chickpeas Wellington 59
    Garbanzo Fritters 37
    Mexican Chickpeas 57
    Sag Madras 64
Chickpeas Provençale 20
Chickpeas Wellington 59

Chilli Beans 85
Chilli Sauce 85
Chilli sin Carne 62
Chinese Vegetables with Pasta 83
Coulis 102
Couscous 102
    Capsicum and Chickpea Couscous 35
"Crisp" Savory Cheesecake 43
Croquettes Mont Blanc 33
Crumble Topping 13
Curry Sauce 97

Dariole mold 102
Delhi Lasagne 10
Dhal 70
Dumplings
    Cheese 71
    Parsley 93

Egg Bombay 68
Eggplant and Zucchini Bake 27
Eggplant Layer 49
Eggplant Parcels 46
Eggs
    Egg Bombay 68
    Omelette Collection 39

Fat 2
Fiber 2
Fillings for sandwiches 101
Filo pastry
    Eggplant Parcels 46
    Filo Pastry Baskets 5
    Spinach Roulade 79
Flageolet beans 4